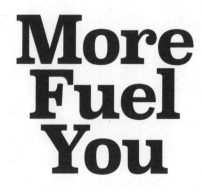

More Fuel You

More Fuel You

UNDERSTANDING YOUR BODY & HOW TO FUEL YOUR ADVENTURES

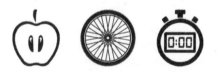

RENEE McGREGOR

Vertebrate Publishing, Sheffield
www.adventurebooks.com

More Fuel You

RENEE McGREGOR

First published in 2022 by Vertebrate Publishing. Reprinted in 2022.

 Vertebrate Publishing
Omega Court, 352 Cemetery Road, Sheffield S11 8FT, United Kingdom.
www.adventurebooks.com

This book is a work of non-fiction. The author has stated to the publishers that, except in such minor respects not affecting the substantial accuracy of the work, the contents of the book are true.

A CIP catalogue record for this book is available from the British Library.

ISBN: 978-1-83981-082-4 (Paperback)
ISBN: 978-1-83981-083-1 (Ebook)
ISBN: 978-1-83981-084-8 (Audiobook)

10 9 8 7 6 5 4 3 2

Edited by Jen Benson.
Cover design by Jane Beagley, Vertebrate Publishing, www.adventurebooks.com
Layout and production by Geoff Borin, www.geoffborinbooks.com

Vertebrate Publishing is committed to printing on paper from sustainable sources.

FSC logo here

Printed and bound in Great Britain by Clays Ltd., Elcograf S.p.A.

To Maya and Ella.

Always believe and shine bright.

CONTENTS

FOREWORD by Damian Hall IX

A WORD FROM THE AUTHOR 1

INTRODUCTION 7

PART 1: **Fuelling for Training and Competition** 11

CHAPTER 1: **Food as Fuel** 13

CHAPTER 2: **Athlete Diets** 52

CHAPTER 3: **Low-Carbohydrate Diets** 56

CHAPTER 4: **Vegan and Plant-Based Diets** 68

CHAPTER 5: **Intermittent Fasting** 78

CHAPTER 6: **Calorie-Controlled Diets** 87

PART 2: **Fuelling for Specific Populations** 101

CHAPTER 7: **The Female Athlete** 103

CHAPTER 8: **The Masters Athlete** 130

CHAPTER 9: **The Individual Athlete** 138

CHAPTER 10: **Over to You** 145

ACKNOWLEDGEMENTS 163

NOTES 165

BIBLIOGRAPHY AND REFERENCES 171

ABOUT THE AUTHOR 180

FOREWORD

Renee and I go back to the misty dawn of time. Well, 2013 anyway, pretty much the start of my ultrarunning career. I was about to do the Spine Race and was semi-certain I was going to die. I can't remember if I asked or if she offered, but I learnt she was a sports dietitian in our local trail-running group, the Bath Bats, and she kindly gave me advice on how to fuel for a 268-mile race in January.

I still remember some of it. Protein shakes would be a smart move at the main checkpoints, she said, plus bagels have more calories/carbs than normal bread. Oh, and try not to die.

Because as well as being a world-renowned expert on various aspects of nutrition, Renee cares too. That's obvious from the areas her work has gone into. In fact, she's probably the busiest person I know. It's been thrilling to watch her career trajectory, from offering advice to green pipsqueaks like me to supporting medal-bothering Olympians and being on the telly a lot. Crucially, along the way she's also helped so many people overcome complex relationships with food and raised awareness for previously invisible issues such as RED-S, which will have helped countless others.

Something worked for me on that first Spine Race, and it probably wasn't just the nut butter bagels that got me to the end. But I've been pestering Renee for advice about the best nosh to stick in my cakehole ever since: for races in the Arctic, the Sahara, for my best runs at UTMB, before setting records on various National Trails.

When unconventional fuelling ideas have gained popularity in the running world, to the point where they've made me curious, I've asked for her thoughts. She's always been strict that she'll only give advice backed by science. But both in person and in writing she delivers it in an accessible way. I think I've only ignored her words of wisdom once – regarding low-carb, high-fat diets – and I regretted that.

As I've accidentally stumbled into confession mode, the idea that 'the lighter a runner, the faster they'll be' was in my mind a few years back and I'm glad Renee talked some sense into me there, too. My best results, and longest spells uninjured, have occurred when I haven't been stepping neurotically on to the scales each day.

Talking of honesty, Renee's is striking and ultimately helps us identify with her and perhaps be more forgiving of ourselves, too. We're all human and life can be tough. But here are some science-backed, easy-to-understand ideas, delivered with compassion, that will help you.

Not only am I still working with Renee nine years later, but we're collaborating more closely than ever. Knowing – and, importantly, following advice from – Renee has helped make me a better athlete and person.

In the same way that a physiotherapist who tells a runner they can still run with a niggle is a keeper, so too is a sports dietitian who not only encourages copious consumption of tea and chocolate milk (though perhaps not together), but who herself eats (dark) chocolate daily.

Damian Hall, record-breaking ultrarunner, coach and author

A WORD FROM THE AUTHOR

Food is such a simple human need: something that should provide us with pleasure and with the energy to live and do the activities that we want, while also being central to our relationships and well-being. But the longer I work in the nutrition industry, the more I notice how far we are straying from these principles, into a global marketplace dominated and controlled by those more interested in making money than nurturing people and communities.

Throughout my career I have worked with numerous individuals from a range of different backgrounds in both the clinical and sports sectors: non-athletes, athletes of all levels, those of all ages, from junior to masters, and across numerous sports. What I find fascinating is that regardless of who I work with, the messages around food are invariably both confusing and confused.

In the twenty years I have been working in the field of nutrition, never have our choices around food been so closely tied to our identities as they are today. What, and how, we eat is about so much more than our food preferences – for many, it is about the message we want to send out to the world, the identity we want to forge for ourselves and present to others. We seem to have lost the art of eating for joy and sustenance somewhere in the confusion of both mainstream and social media messaging. Add wearable tech and food-tracking apps into the mix, each of which is designed with its own set of agendas, and it's hardly surprising that we are coming to rely on external cues for choosing what, and when, to eat, rather than our fantastically complex internal monitoring systems, which really are based on what our body needs.

Working with athletes is not just about improving and optimising performance outcomes; it is also about helping people to adopt a healthy attitude and balance in their relationship with food. Surrounded by mixed messages and poorly researched information, it is hardly surprising that many aspiring athletes – both at recreational and elite levels – struggle with this balance. If we're not careful, the constant need to follow the most up-to-date diet as recommended by the latest social media sensation can lead to poorly informed decisions, and this is doubtless fuelling the current rise in dysfunctional relationships with eating. Tying our dietary choices up with our sense of worth, whether that's feeling virtuous about veganism or believing that we need to 'earn' our food before we're allowed to eat it, cannot provide the foundation for a good relationship. It makes me sad to watch as food seems to have become the enemy rather than something that brings joy.

So, when Vertebrate asked me to write this book, I didn't need to consider it. It was the book I wanted to write. I have always been told that what makes me good at my job is the ability to cut through the bullshit and make the science both practical and accessible to all. I wanted to write a book that provided individuals with the facts all in one place so that they could go on to make an informed choice about how they would like to eat, devoid of judgement. Moreover, I wanted to bring the fun and joy back to eating, while still helping people meet their fuelling requirements.

* * *

My own journey with food is one with many twists and turns, influenced hugely by my childhood, the places I have travelled, my job and of course my own personal experience of fuelling my running adventures.

My parents are Indian, Punjabi Sikh to be precise, and they moved to the UK in the mid-1960s after an arranged marriage. Settling in London, they did all they could to source traditional ingredients so that they could maintain the diet they were not only familiar with, but that provided huge comfort when becoming accustomed to a foreign land. I was born ten years after they arrived in the UK and for the first few years of my life, prior to attending school, I was brought up on a diet of rice, chapatis, lentils and vegetable curries. Food is really important in Indian families – it is very much the heart of the home. My earliest memories of food are of eating together, enjoying the vast array of flavours, surrounded by conversation and laughter.

My parents were vegetarian and, although they never insisted I follow in their footsteps, I have chosen to remain vegetarian, mainly because I don't like the taste of meat. I find it interesting that, while my diet is very varied now, I still have a big preference for spicy foods and always favour a curry over a burger or fish and chips, which backs up the idea that our early food experiences hugely impact our preferences in adult life.

It was only once I started school that the curiosity of how others ate, plus the desire to be accepted by my peers, made our diet as a family slowly start to change and include more Western cuisine. School lunches were definitely not much to write home about, but once I started being invited to friends' houses, going to parties and attending Brownies, my journey of exploration with different foods and traditions gradually grew, paving the way for how I eat today.

I have many wonderful memories around food, but the one that always comes to mind is the first time I was introduced to the baked potato. I remember it clearly even now, nearly forty years later. I was six years old and we had been invited to our neighbours' for Bonfire Night. I was so excited because we had never been to a bonfire gathering before. While I was familiar with fireworks from our annual Diwali celebrations, this was something different, and it was even more exciting as we had been learning about Guy Fawkes at school. As we stood there amongst the oohs and aahs, we were handed small, foil-wrapped packages; they were like precious gifts and, boy, did they bring joy. I will never forget that first mouthful of hot potato mixed with melted butter and cheese. It was absolutely delicious and, to this day, baked potatoes are a firm favourite and regularly appear on my menu. This memory is hugely significant for me. It created such a positive association with the act of nourishing my body, which in my mind is a big part of the role of food in our lives.

Sadly, my relationship with food was not always so easy. During my teenage years, not eating became a way of punishing myself for feeling as though I wasn't good enough. I didn't feel accepted by my peers or the society that I had been born into. The colour of my skin didn't fit, I didn't fit and, subsequently, I wanted to become as small and insignificant as I felt. Avoiding or 'containing' food provided a false sense of security, a coping mechanism, a method of denying those difficult and traumatic emotions I was not prepared for, or even mature enough to face at that stage. Thankfully, I eventually did tackle and overcome those difficulties and, though traumatic at the time, my past experiences provide an essential insight into my practice today.

Becoming a dietitian and spending eight years working in the NHS has also had a big impact on my relationship with food. As well as arming me with the knowledge and understanding to underpin my own nutrition, working with many unwell patients who were often desperate to eat but unable to do so due to a wide range of clinical problems finally helped me to fully appreciate and be grateful for the joys of eating. While I no longer work in the NHS, I will always see it as being paramount to my career journey. I learnt to be flexible and adaptable, and to think on my feet. I learnt that, while knowing the theory was essential, humans are not textbooks and often have multiple issues occurring at the same time. These experiences helped me to become more resourceful and provided the best grounding and platform to grow from. More recently, I have learnt so much from spending time in places like Nepal, a country that not only stole my heart but showed me how lucky we are in the Western world where we take running water and food availability for granted.

By the time I left the NHS, I was also a mum to young daughters. Becoming a parent changed my entire outlook on life. I felt a huge sense of responsibility – not just to provide my children's growing bodies with good nourishment, but also to nurture their sense of worth, develop their self-confidence, and help them navigate life and all that it brings with it. Through both my professional and personal experiences, my aim has always been to try to be a good role model.

For this reason, we never talk about 'good' or 'bad' foods at home, but instead about eating some foods less often. Being physically active is about fun and enjoyment, not achieving a particular body size or excelling in a given sport. And, most importantly, I want my daughters to grow up knowing that they are not defined by their looks or their achievements, but loved and accepted for who they are, with the onus on appreciating that we don't fail, but we learn and gain knowledge from every experience, which in turn creates more opportunity. I guess in some way, it is these values that have also helped me to progress in my career and in turn help others.

The move into sports nutrition seemed like a logical step to me. I had always been a sporty child – I swam, danced, played hockey and netball. Being physically active is something that gave me, and still does give me, huge pleasure. So, while the girls were still young and at home, I set about completing my second postgraduate qualification, this time in applied sports nutrition. What came next has been a diverse career spanning more than ten years working with a real mix of athletes, attendance at major international competitions, including the Rio 2016 Paralympics, and input into numerous nutritional protocols and pathways within various sporting organisations.

I got into running when my youngest daughter was eleven months old as a means of creating a small window for myself and allowing Mother Nature to do what she did best and help lift my mood. I was struggling with postnatal depression and my twenty-minute run a few times a week made a big difference. Since then, I have built my mileage up slowly and moved up from half marathon to marathon, from road to trail, to where I am now, running ultramarathons over a mix of terrains but with a real love for mountain and forest trails. While I don't think it is necessarily a prerequisite for practice, I do think my own experiences in endurance sport help me to understand those of the athletes I work with better.

As for me, I still don't always get it right and I have made my fair share of mistakes along the way. When I started running, even though I had the knowledge, I don't think I fully trusted or appreciated just how much energy it took to be able to run consistently well and progress. I fell into the trap of worrying about undoing all the good of training by eating too much and subsequently can see that, while it was accidental, I did under-fuel for a long time. Restoring a healthy balance brought its rewards to both my running and my health.

People are often curious about my relationship with food and training. I can hand on heart say that I now eat to train rather than train to eat. Eating in this way has not only made food enjoyable again but has significantly improved my performance and allowed me to train consistently, even as I get older. Like any long-term relationship, my relationship with food has had many twists and turns along the way, but through experience, both professional and personal, I finally feel like I have a great attitude towards eating, and it is exactly this which I hope you will all gain from reading this book.

INTRODUCTION

The idea that nutrition and performance are inextricably linked is not new, but knowledge around the topic is growing and evolving all the time. The first scientific studies on carbohydrate and fat metabolism in athletes were conducted in Sweden in the 1930s, igniting an interest in diet as a performance aid. Since then, sports nutrition has become a standalone science, with many diverse branches and specialisms emerging over the years.

While well-conducted scientific research is essential for understanding and advancing the field of sports nutrition, interpreting its findings isn't always straightforward. Studies are often hard to access in full, inaccurately reported by the mass media, or they use a very specific group of participants, making them less relevant to the wider population. A study involving male trained athletes that looks at nutritional needs at altitude, for example, is not necessarily going to be relevant for untrained males, any female athletes, or those training at sea level.

So where else can we go for information and advice on the best way to eat to fuel our training? Social media is a relatively recent phenomenon, and yet it is already hugely influential in shaping the lives – and food choices – of many. A study from Aston University in 2020 demonstrated that other people can have a huge influence over our food choices, concluding that:

> 'We may be influenced by our social peers more than we realize when choosing certain foods; we seem to be subconsciously accounting for how others behave when making our own food choices.'[1]

Indeed, we have to appreciate that nutrition in general, regardless of whether it is sports-related or not, is a highly personal and individual experience. Nutrition is multi-faceted, in that it is not just about the nutrients we put in our bodies, but also about the role it plays in our lifestyles, as well as the psychology involved.

How we choose what we eat is influenced by many factors, which differ between people and also for any individual from one day to the next.

They include:

- hunger and preference
- education
- budget, income and food availability
- cultural beliefs, family, peers and habits
- mood, stress and guilt
- media and social media
- food trends
- supermarkets/offers
- attitudes, beliefs and relationship with self.

Additionally, we cannot forget that food choice is important because it creates consumer demand for suppliers who produce, process and distribute food.[2] The global sports nutrition market was valued at 50.84 billion US dollars in 2018 and is expected to increase to 81.5 billion US dollars by 2023.[3] It is clear that big businesses have a lot to gain by using influential personalities to promote their products. While some sports nutrition products may have a part to play in optimal performance, most are just an expensive gimmick. If it sounds too good to be true, then it probably is too good to be true; in reality, there are never any quick fixes when it comes to nutrition, health or performance.

We live in an age where anyone can set themselves up as an expert and reach millions without any relevant qualifications or experience and in a mostly unregulated space – sadly with potentially disastrous consequences for their followers. The rise and fall of the 'clean eating' movement is a good example of widely accepted nutritional advice devoid of scientific or expert input. In the field of sports nutrition, the allure of fad diets also extends to their proposed performance benefits. Whether your aim is to get leaner, stronger or faster, to bulk up or drop weight fast, someone has a diet that guarantees success.

There is no doubt that what we eat has a huge impact on both our physical and mental health and well-being, and on our performance when it comes to training for, and competing in, our chosen sport. So how do we navigate the maze of conflicting information out there, choose a way of eating that is right for us, and make sure we do it as well as possible? That's where this book can help.

In the first part of this book, I aim to address each of the most popular athlete diets around today: what they are, how they work and how to approach them safely, with optimal health and performance in mind. I guide you through the key points you need to know, and the dangers and pitfalls to look out for as you go. In the second part, the focus is on population groups that are often overlooked in the sports nutrition world, where research is scant but the importance of good fuelling is still highly significant. Throughout the book, I have included authentic case studies, each of which retains the individual athlete's own words.

For simplicity, I'm going to use the term 'athlete' for all levels and abilities in sport. So, whether you're a runner, cyclist or climber, recreational, professional or elite level, you'll discover how to eat best for you and your sport based on both the most up-to-date science and my twenty years of experience as a dietitian and sports nutritionist.

PART 1

Fuelling for Training and Competition

In this first part of the book, we explore energy requirements, look at what informs our food choice, and deep-dive into some of the more popular nutrition approaches and trends followed by athletes.

CHAPTER 1

Food as Fuel

Sports nutrition: the basics

From a physiological perspective, the basic role of the food we eat is to provide both the energy and nutrients we need to fuel our bodies in the form of the three macronutrients – carbohydrates, fats and proteins – and the micronutrients essential for optimal functioning and health. Once eaten, digested and absorbed, the energy from food needs to be converted into a form that is usable for powering our activities: adenosine triphosphate (ATP). ATP is produced in our mitochondria – the powerhouses of our cells – providing energy through three different pathways:

1 The immediate energy system (or ATP-PCr), which utilises stored ATP for explosive bouts of activity lasting less than 10 seconds, such as jumping over a stream or out of the way of a car. The supply of ATP in this system is highly limited, but extremely useful for fight-or-flight situations when there is no time to wait for the production of ATP via the two other pathways.

2 The lactic acid (or anaerobic) system, which provides rapid energy for intensive activity such as running up a hill, sprinting for the finish line or making a short but powerful series of moves on the climbing wall. Using carbohydrate as a fuel, this system produces ATP by converting glucose molecules into lactate which, while faster than the aerobic system described below, is less efficient and produces the metabolites responsible for the infamous lactate 'burn'.

3 The aerobic system, which is responsible for the majority of our energy production for daily life. It is highly flexible, is able to utilise all the macronutrients as fuel, and is by far the most efficient system, producing the most ATP per glucose molecule, with only carbon dioxide and water as waste products.

While it's tempting to see our energy systems as separate entities with different roles, in reality they all work together constantly, with each one being brought to the fore when it is required and the others continuing to work in the background.

These principles are the same for everyone, regardless of athletic undertaking; and the energy derived from foods, regardless of the type of food it originally came from, is utilised in the same way. And yet, as introduced in the previous section, the world of nutrition is a complex and often quite emotive subject, and one we are bombarded with messages about on a daily basis. Additionally, as individuals, each with our own set of specific requirements, no one approach is going to be suitable for all. So, when faced with so much – often conflicting – advice on the topic, where do we start?

As athletes, it's important to remember that an optimal diet must be adequate to support our health, our daily life and our chosen sport. So how does an athlete diet differ from one recommended for more sedentary people?

While the two are not entirely separate entities, the specific role of nutrition in sport takes in the following factors:

Fuelling and recovery

The best-known role of nutrition is to fuel the body ready for training, and in response to training as adaptation and recovery. Sufficient energy from our diet is essential both for the healthy functioning of our bodies and for physical activity and, throughout this book, is referred to in kilocalories (kcal or Cal, equal to 1,000 calories). Recommendations for energy intake are given as kilocalories per kilogram of body weight.

The composition and timing of what we eat are critical to support training, but also to allow for optimal adaptation from the training stimulus, resulting in overall, consistent progression.

Body composition

The term 'body composition' refers to a person's ratio of lean tissue (muscle) to fat tissue mass. Optimal body composition varies widely from person to person and between sports. But, as a general rule, if you make sensible, well-informed choices around nutrition and training load – in particular the composition, timing and amounts of food – your body will respond and adapt accordingly, resulting in an appropriate body composition for both you and your sport. This latter point is really important as, while many sports may project certain body ideals, factors such as genetics, gender and our phenotype (the observable results of the combination of our genetics and environment, for example our appearance, development and behaviour) all play a role in determining what is a realistic, healthy and optimal body composition for us as individuals.

Bone health

The strength, density and architecture of our bones are important for sport and for long-term health and quality of life. Most people reach their peak bone mass – their highest level of bone mineral density – between the ages of twenty-five and thirty, a process influenced by both genetic and lifestyle factors. Our bones respond to the stimuli exerted upon them, modelling and remodelling in response to the magnitude and direction of forces. Physical activity, in particular weightbearing forms such as running, walking and some resistance training, along with good nutrition, have an important role to play in building and maintaining our bone health, especially as it starts to decline naturally from our forties onwards. While most people assume that doing exercise automatically supports optimal bone health, sports such as cycling, swimming and rowing are not sufficiently weightbearing to do this. Climbing, depending on what discipline is undertaken, may include both weightbearing and non-weightbearing elements. Ensuring that both weightbearing and resistance exercise is incorporated into a training programme, and that all exercise is supported by a diet that meets both nutritional and energy needs, is essential for maintaining good bone health.

A diet providing a suitable energy intake along with key nutrients, vitamin D and calcium also supports optimal levels of the sex hormones oestrogen and testosterone, which play a critical role in maintaining bone health, something we'll discuss in greater detail later.

Dual-energy X-ray absorptiometry (DXA) is the gold standard for measuring bone mineral density. It is commonly used for diagnosing osteopenia (lower than normal bone density) and osteoporosis (severe loss of bone mineral density and bone mass, or structural changes in the bone), for monitoring changes in bone density over time, and for assessing fracture risk. When interpreting the findings of a DXA scan, it is essential to take into account the full range of an individual's characteristics, from age and ethnicity to body size and training history, before drawing conclusions and making recommendations. Based on ethnic background alone, for example, people of Afro–Caribbean heritage have, on average, a higher bone density than people of Caucasian or Asian heritage. People with a naturally smaller body size will have a lower bone density compared with naturally larger, heavier individuals. And, as we get older, due to declining testosterone and oestrogen levels, we also start to see a decline in bone density, a key consideration for masters athletes, which is discussed further in chapter 8.

Consistency in training

While fitness trends come and go, being able to maintain consistency in training is what results in optimal athletic performance. Most of us who take part in sport know that when we can complete a training block without interruption through injury, illness or other lifestyle factors, we tend to see our best results. Nutrition plays a vital role in this, too. Meeting your nutritional requirements gives your body the fuel to perform and recover optimally. Adequate nutritional intake also supports the immune system, reducing risk of illness.

Mood and motivation

Good nutrition and adequate recovery are also essential in supporting our motivation to train and overall mood. We know that a certain amount of functional fatigue is important to drive adaptation from training. But, while it is normal to have the odd day when it's a struggle to get out of bed to train, especially midway through a heavy training block, frequent or longer-lasting bouts of fatigue and low motivation, or prolonged irritability and low mood, could indicate a chronic lack of recovery and/or insufficient fuelling.

Injury and illness risk

Ensuring sufficient overall energy intake, with a particular focus on carbohydrate availability around training, supports optimal progression in training, but also helps to prevent the immune system from becoming compromised, reducing the risk of illness. Similarly, a well-fuelled body is less likely to incur injuries related to overreaching or poor recovery.

Hormonal and biochemical regulation

A raft of different hormones drives and regulates biological processes within our bodies, including our reproductive systems, our metabolic rate and our body composition. However, hormones can only work effectively if there is sufficient energy in the system. Ensuring adequate and appropriate nutrition around training is critical for hormonal regulation and optimal health and performance.

The key role of hormones in all these processes is often overlooked, especially in female athletes. While we have ample evidence of the role of testosterone when it comes to body composition, strength and speed,

MORE FUEL YOU

little attention is given to oestrogen. Oestrogen, like testosterone, is a sex hormone but has multiple roles within the body, including menstruation, bone health, cognitive function and body composition. Thus, maintaining oestrogen at an appropriate level is essential for optimal performance in females. We will discuss this in a lot more detail in the second part of this book.

When athletes come to my clinic, I often use blood testing to check for certain markers that help me identify if an athlete has any nutritional deficiencies, is recovering appropriately and is meeting their energy requirements. However, I appreciate that not everyone can – or wants to – undertake regular blood tests, and interpreting results appropriately for the specific requirements of athletes can be difficult, even for medical professionals. Fortunately, as humans, we are actually very good at assessing how we feel subjectively, a fact it is important not to overlook in a world of wearable technology, metrics and data.

While such tangible data can, when interpreted in the right way, be helpful in assessing the overall picture of an athlete, of which diet is an important part, most are composite scores based on approximations and averages. It is important, therefore, to always consider them alongside the key piece of data that only you really know: how you feel. Training should be enjoyable – something you want to do, rather than feel you have to do. Feeling hungry and thinking about food constantly; fatigue, low motivation and mood; low libido or reproductive dysfunction; and frequent or unusual muscle soreness may all indicate either a deficiency of certain nutrients, poor recovery or a lack of overall energy in your diet. If these symptoms become persistent or chronic, they should not be ignored and should be investigated by a qualified practitioner.

The section above outlines the many and varied roles of sports nutrition in both health and performance. But a question I'm often asked is how the approach to sports nutrition differs for recreational athletes compared with those of an elite or professional level. The answer is that the general principles apply to anyone who is participating in a sporting activity, regardless of their level. The athletes I work with want to achieve the best possible outcome for their individual set of circumstances. While for the elites this may be more focused on achieving a specific time or podium placing, for recreational athletes it may be more about getting to the finish line and simply completing a challenge. Either way, it is the same set of metabolic principles that underpin my advice and guidance.

The next section outlines the key nutrients and biological processes applicable to all, and how these all piece together, for optimal health but also, specifically when it comes to training and competing, to help you achieve your desired performance outcome.

Calculating energy expenditure

The human body is a fantastically complex organism featuring a number of distinct and yet interdependent biological systems, each of which contributes in its own way to the overall conditions necessary for everyday living. These systems include:

- The cardiovascular system, responsible for blood circulation around the body, delivering oxygen and nutrients to cells, and removing waste products.
- The respiratory system, divided into the upper and lower respiratory tract, jointly responsible for absorbing oxygen and removing carbon dioxide via gaseous exchange in the lungs.
- The digestive system, responsible for processing the food we eat, absorbing fuel and nutrients, and removing waste products.
- The endocrine system – the body's messenger system – responsible for monitoring and releasing regulatory hormones under the overall control of the hypothalamus in the brain.
- The integumentary system – the barrier against the external environment formed by our skin, along with our hair and nails – which detects external stimuli and protects the body's internal environment.

- The immune (or lymphatic) system, which detects and responds to potential threats from pathogens such as bacteria and viruses.
- The musculoskeletal system – the body's bony architecture, providing structure, support and protection, and the muscles that permit movement.
- The nervous system, comprising the central nervous system (the CNS – the brain and spinal cord) and the peripheral nervous system (the PNS – the nerves connecting the CNS to every other part of the body).
- The renal system, which eliminates waste from the body, regulates the volume, pressure and pH of the blood, and controls levels of electrolytes and metabolites.
- The reproductive system – the organs and associated processes involved in sexual reproduction.

Before any level of activity has begun, all of these systems require energy simply to keep us alive and healthy. Our basal metabolic rate (BMR, also known as our resting metabolic rate or RMR) is an estimate of the energy requirement for the resting body, lying down in the early morning with an empty stomach and at a comfortable temperature. BMR increases with body weight and differs between individuals of different ages and sexes, but is responsible for 60–75% of energy requirements in sedentary individuals.

On top of the energy required for basal metabolism, the thermic effect of feeding (TEF) is the energy used to digest food, and can be 10–20% of our total energy requirements. Finally, there is the thermic effect of activity (TEA), which is the energy utilised by our body for movement, including training. This is heavily influenced by the type, duration and intensity of exercise and can be as high as an additional 70% in elite athletes, but usually sits around 25–50% in recreational athletes, and up to 25% of those who are sedentary. It is important to appreciate that TEA is the energy cost of all movement, not just training, so will include everything from getting out of bed and brushing your teeth to shopping, housework and walking the dog.

A key element of good sports nutrition is to ensure there is sufficient energy availability (EA) for the basic functions of the body once the energy required for physical activity has been deducted from overall energy intake. Long-term insufficient fuelling resulting in a lack of available energy remaining for the functioning, repair and maintenance of the body after exercise can lead to a condition known as relative energy deficiency in sport (RED-S), which will be discussed in greater detail later.

With so many variables to take into account, how can we calculate an accurate figure for energy expenditure? Adding together the above values can give us a rough estimate of overall energy requirements, but the human body is well adapted for survival in widely varying conditions, sparing energy in times of low food availability and maximising storage as body fat when supplies are plentiful. Some people, such as children, smaller-than-average adults and those with a high percentage of lean mass, burn more energy than expected, while others burn less. As a result, particularly with active individuals, calculating energy requirements accurately is difficult, particularly outside of a lab-based environment. And even once an estimate of overall energy requirements has been calculated, this does not address the specific balance of macronutrients – carbohydrates, fats and proteins – needed to support exercise and training.

It's easy to see why many athletes rely on wearable technology and apps to record and calculate energy requirements. However, it is important to appreciate that these algorithms can only ever estimate the real figures and in many cases may be inaccurate, while giving us very little information about the composition of the diet or the optimal nutrient timing to help with our performance goals. Even the way in which information is gathered and utilised is questionable – I find that I often hit 10,000 steps a day when I'm driving!

Based on cues of hunger and satiety, athletes themselves are often a good gauge of how much they need to eat to meet their energy requirements, and a well-balanced and varied diet should provide adequate nutritional requirements. However, particularly during times of heavy training, or when striving for a body composition, weight or performance goal, even this approach – often referred to as intuitive eating – may not be sufficient for optimal health and performance.

It can also be difficult to calculate energy expenditure over a variety of different activities, both sporting and otherwise, a figure which is likely to vary day to day. Even the energy used for individual sports varies widely depending upon the duration, intensity and specific conditions of that session. A good example is comparing the energy cost of indoor climbing with running at a steady state, so around a perceived effort of around seven out of ten. In a 60-kilogram athlete, both will cost around 11 kilocalories per minute of activity. While running may be more continuous, climbing still demands a lot of energy for each move. The two sports rely predominantly on different energy systems that both yield high amounts of energy. Endurance running relies more heavily on the aerobic system, which can provide a more continuous form of energy to the muscles as long as there is adequate oxygen and fuel available; whereas climbing, while it does use the aerobic system, also utilises the immediate energy and anaerobic systems to provide bursts of energy over very short time frames. This is the case in most sports, where all three energy pathways will be engaged but in different combinations. The anaerobic system needs more time to recover between movements but can support repeated movements over time, whereas the aerobic system supports more continuous delivery of energy to the working muscles. There's a common misconception that more energy is utilised in endurance sports, but this example shows us that when you compare minute to minute, the overall energy use for the session is the same.

Added to all these factors are the changes in our BMR that occur in the immediate post-exercise phase, allowing us to recover and adapt ready for the next bout of exercise. It's easy to see how relying on algorithms or even calculations based on basic 'energy in' versus 'energy out' assumptions can often fall short. As we said right at the start of this section, humans are not textbooks, and being fully aware of the individuality of both our bodies and our lifestyles is essential in order to fuel for optimal health and performance.

The information which follows has come from the scientific literature available on the active population, but I can't stress enough that this *is still an estimation* and doesn't take into consideration the breakdown of macronutrients required for optimal performance, adaptation and progression. These are areas to be worked out on an individual basis, either through careful monitoring of the above measures (such as mood and motivation, progression in training and immune health), or by working with a qualified professional.

As we discussed above, in active people, energy availability (EA) – the available energy to maintain body processes once the energy required for physical activity has been accounted for – is essential for optimal health, and therefore long-term athletic performance. When calculating values for EA for sports nutrition purposes, we typically use kilocalories per kilogram of fat-free mass (FFM), where FFM is everything our body is composed of other than fat. The reason we use FFM rather than overall body mass is because bodies with a higher percentage of fat typically require less energy per kilogram than bodies with a lower percentage of fat, as, even at rest, muscle cells burn more energy than fat cells.

The only way to get a true measure of your FFM is by having a DXA scan or skinfold measurement by an experienced practitioner, but we can estimate FFM based on overall body mass and where on the spectrum of low to high body-fat percentage you currently reside. As an example, for a lean, 60-kilogram athlete, a typical FFM might be around 47 kilograms, with a fat mass of 13 kilograms (about 22% body fat). Another athlete with the same body mass of 60 kilograms but with a fat mass of 20 kilograms (about 33% body fat) will have a FFM of 40 kilograms. An energy availability calculation (see overleaf) would result in different outcomes, even though both athletes have the same body mass – a good illustration of the pitfalls of calculating energy requirements based upon body mass alone.

GENERAL 'ATHLETIC' REQUIREMENTS

- Energy availability (EA) should never drop below 35 kilocalories per kilogram of FFM to ensure optimal health.

- In female athletes who train at a moderate intensity for 60–90 minutes a day, EA should be 45–50 kilocalories per kilogram of FFM.

- In male athletes who train at a moderate intensity for 60–90 minutes a day, EA requirements are more than 50 kilocalories per kilogram of FFM.

Using these recommendations to estimate the energy availability of a 60-kilogram female athlete who climbs for a maximum of ninety minutes a day and has 22% body fat:

22% of 60 kilograms is just over 13 kilograms

60 − 13 = 47 kilograms of FFM

Let's say she consumes 2,700 calories during this day but burns 990 calories (11 calories per minute) through her climbing, plus an additional 300 calories through daily movement. This then leaves 1,410 calories. If we divide this by 47 kilograms, her FFM, to give us a value of kilocalories per kilogram, EA is 30 kilocalories per kilogram of FFM, so under the minimal amount needed to support biological function.

If we use the same method but for an athlete who has a lower FFM (40 kilograms), EA would be 35 kilocalories per kilogram and in this case would support biological function.

Thus, our climber's energy requirements are not just determined by the amount of training she does but also by her body composition. Additionally, you can see how important it is to include other energy requirements, the highest of which is usually non-sporting physical activity. For athletes who commute on foot or by bike, have an active job, walk the dog or run around after small children, the real figure could be substantially higher than this. And all that is before we explore the challenges involved in determining the energy value of different foods – how can we make sure we're fuelling ourselves with the right amount of energy?

Calculating energy intake

One of the reasons I studied biochemistry as an undergraduate was that the human body fascinated me. I wanted to understand how it all came together. What did it take to make this incredible vessel work effectively? What allowed it to be so resilient and adaptable to both internal and external stressors? One of the most intriguing discoveries I made was that the 'Calories in' versus 'Calories out' model, based on published Calorie values of different foods, was deeply flawed. And this is why.

All foods yield energy, usually measured in the form of Calories (note the capital 'C', which represents 1,000 calories and is also referred to as a kilocalorie or kcal, where one kilocalorie is the energy required to raise one kilogram of water through one degree Celsius). However, different foods, and the various ways they are prepared, impact our bodies in different ways.

For example, if we were to burn 200 grams of carrots in a calorimeter (the original method used to ascertain the energy value of foods), this would yield an energy value in kilocalories. While this will be low, we might assume that we will absorb all these calories but, due to the high fibre content of carrots, very little of the energy from a carrot is available to be utilised by our bodies as energy. Processing foods, for example cooking carrots to break down some of the indigestible fibre, increases the amount of energy we can extract from them. The kilocalories in highly processed foods, on the other hand, are easily and rapidly absorbed. So 100 kilocalories' worth of raw carrot and 100 kilocalories' worth of jelly babies will have very different effects on the body, with the jelly babies being easily and completely digested and absorbed (making them an ideal choice for consuming on the run) compared with the carrots, which demand more work to be done to extract their available energy. In addition to their easy Calories, highly processed foods commonly have a low nutrient value and are very easy to consume without causing satiety – tricking our brains into believing we are not yet full – so they are also very easy to overconsume. It is not these foods in isolation that will cause us to gain weight, it is more the fact that they are easy to consume and provide very little nutritional benefit to the body.

Like other living organisms, the internal conditions of the human body are carefully monitored and controlled to keep them working optimally – a process called homeostasis. Deviations away from optimal conditions are quickly detected by the body's monitoring systems, and action is taken to restore them. Examples well known to athletes are shivering or sweating to control body temperature, thirst and urination to control water content, and varying breathing rates to control oxygen and carbon dioxide levels. Blood glucose levels are another variable under close homeostatic control. The glucose derived from our diets is essential for cell respiration – the process that produces energy for everything from basic processes to athletic performance, discussed above. When we eat, causing blood glucose levels to rise, insulin is released from the pancreas, which stimulates uptake of glucose into the liver and muscle cells until blood glucose levels return to normal. When blood glucose levels fall, insulin secretion reduces, resulting in a reduction in glucose uptake from the blood and again restoring levels to normal.

It is these same intricate connections and systems in the body that also make weight loss so difficult. We know that to maintain weight we need to be in energy balance – that is, our energy intake is in equilibrium with our energy output. This has then led to the belief that if we reduce energy input but increase energy output, we will lose weight, and vice versa. However, it really isn't as simple as that. This is because human physiology is biased towards maintaining energy balance, and this works best at higher levels of energy intake and expenditure – that is, to have a healthy body, we need to move a lot but also take in enough energy to maintain this balance.

Our physiology has evolved to maintain this energy balance even in times of low food availability, protecting us against starvation, which would once have been a reality of human life. We store fat readily when we take in more energy than we expend. But weight loss, when it does occur, triggers compensatory decreases in energy expenditure that generally facilitate weight regain. Therefore, diets in general, and particularly very low-calorie interventions in obese populations, are rarely successful. When we lose weight, our metabolic rate slows, meaning even at rest we burn fewer calories as our bodies attempt to restore that lost weight. What research does show us is that interventions that advocate small changes, as little as an overall deficit of 100 kilocalories a day, have much more promising results, preventing weight regain in most people. This is because the specific components of energy balance influence each other to achieve a constant body mass.

When calorie intake is low, the body responds by stimulating hunger, but also reduces resting metabolic rate so that less energy is expended. Similarly, if we increase energy expenditure, this results in increased hunger as well as reducing the amount of physical activity at other times of the day. For those who want to lose weight, it's easy to believe that it's simply about eating less and moving more, but in reality, our physiology, fine-tuned for survival over hundreds of thousands of years, works against us in a world of abundant food availability.

The components of an athlete diet

Fundamentally, an athlete diet should include all the key components of a normal healthy, balanced diet, combining sufficient energy with the necessary micronutrients for both health and performance. However, sports science research has demonstrated that nutrient timing, overall volume and composition of the diet will vary slightly for athletes from those who are predominantly sedentary, to optimise both training and the subsequent recovery from and adaptation to that training.

As we touched on earlier in this chapter, the food we eat is made up of the three macronutrients: carbohydrate, fat and protein. While many sources might group common foods into only one of these macronutrient categories, in reality the vast majority of foods we eat are composed of a combination of the three, with one often being the most dominant. For example, 100 grams of wholemeal bread contains around 42 grams of carbohydrate, 9 grams of protein and 3 grams of fat; while 100 grams of natural yoghurt contains around 6 grams of carbohydrate, 5 grams of protein and 4 grams of fat. Similarly, our bodies are constantly burning all three macronutrients, to different extents depending on the activity we are undertaking and how rapidly we need energy. When sitting still and reading a book, for example, the body will be mostly burning fat for fuel, although the brain is using carbohydrate. As exercise intensity increases, our bodies increase their burning of both fat and carbohydrate for energy, but the balance shifts more in favour of carbohydrate as it is a quicker and more efficient (although also more limited) source of energy.

So what are the roles of the macronutrients in our diets, both for health and performance?

Carbohydrate

Carbohydrate is the key fuel source for exercise as it is most easily broken down into glucose, the body's preferred source of energy. Carbohydrate is stored as glycogen, primarily within the liver and muscles, with stored muscle glycogen providing ready fuel for physical activity. However, this storage facility is limited.

It takes around 500 grams of carbohydrate to have completely full glycogen stores, about 1,600–2,000 calories' worth, or enough to last for up to about 120 minutes' training at around 65–75% of your maximal heart rate. The harder you work, the faster your stores will deplete; and the more often you train, the more often glycogen stores will be called upon. It is therefore important to plan carbohydrate intake around training sessions; the amount you require will be dependent on the frequency, duration and intensity of your training. A good rule of thumb for endurance activities lasting more than ninety minutes is to aim to take on 60–90 grams per hour, depending on body weight. The amount of carbohydrates a person is able to absorb can be increased a little through training and combining the types of carbohydrate taken in.

Chronically low glycogen stores and insufficient carbohydrate intakes can lead to impaired recovery, increased injury risk and poor performance, making consistency in training more difficult. Carbohydrate availability is also essential for many biological processes, including bone maintenance, hormone regulation – in particular, metabolism-regulating thyroid hormones – and optimal brain function. Our brains make up about 2% of our body weight but consume 20% of our overall energy intake, predominantly derived from glucose. This translates to around 120–130 grams of glucose (400–500 kilocalories) per day. Many sports require the ability to make decisions, whether that is taking the right route when running on the trails, making the next move in climbing or choosing when to overtake in a cycling sportive. If there is not sufficient glucose going to the brain, these decisions become harder to make. Furthermore, the importance of glucose availability in the brain has been demonstrated in studies that look at fatigue of the central nervous system during exercise, with some studies finding that even just taking a mouth swill of glucose in the form of a sports drink can trick the brain into thinking glucose is available, and for a short period of time the individual can maintain their intensity of exercise without taking on actual fuel.[4]

Carbohydrates are formed from chains of molecules containing carbon, hydrogen and oxygen. Complex carbohydrates are the starchier kind, formed from longer chains of carbohydrate molecules that take longer to digest and absorb, including wholegrain pasta, brown rice, oats, couscous, potatoes, wholemeal bread and some cereals. Simple carbohydrates, formed from shorter chains of carbohydrate molecules, are rapidly digested and absorbed, and include sugars found in dairy products, fruit, honey and table sugar, as well as sports drinks.

Physically active people need a mix of both complex and simple carbohydrates – ideally complex carbohydrates at mealtimes and then more simple options immediately before, during and after, depending on the training session.

Some of you may be reading this and thinking, 'But don't carbohydrates make you put on weight?'

In recent years, there has been a plethora of mixed and confusing messages about carbohydrate, leading many people to believe that it is the root cause of weight gain in the Western world. But is it really carbohydrates per se that are the problem? As discussed earlier, we constantly burn both carbs and fat, with fat providing the majority of energy at times of low demand, such as sitting at a desk, and carbs taking over as the main source of energy for higher-intensity activity. But, if we consume more calories than our body needs, any excess will be stored as fat, whether this excess comes from carbohydrate, protein or fat sources. However, it is also important to point out here that it is the balance over several days, weeks and months, not just one day.

Perhaps the confusion lies in the fact that it is quite easy to over-consume carbohydrates, especially if they come in the form of non-nutrient-dense varieties such as drinks and sweets, but also when combined with fat in the case of many baked goods.

Fuelling up with nutrient-dense, complex carbohydrates far ahead enough of activity to allow time for digestion allows glycogen stores to be fully replenished. As we said earlier in the chapter, these stores last for a maximum of about 120 minutes, depending on exercise intensity, and, for longer sessions, can be topped up by ingesting simple carbohydrates. This is where foods such as jelly babies, dried fruits, energy drinks, jam sandwiches made with white bread or energy gels can be very useful. Immediately after exercise it's also important to start replenishing glycogen stores, and this is the ideal time to consume something like flavoured milk, which is high in easily digestible carbohydrates and also in protein to help with recovery.

Carbohydrate requirements

Carbohydrate requirements vary widely depending on the type, duration and intensity of exercise.

- For low-intensity or rest days, requirements are around 3 grams of carbohydrate per kilogram of body weight per day.
- For an hour of moderate training a day, requirements are around 5–7 grams per kilogram of body weight per day.
- For training 1–3 hours a day, requirements are 6–10 grams per kilogram of body weight per day.
- For those training 4–6 hours a day over multiple sessions, requirements are 8–12 grams per kilogram of body weight per day.

But what does this look like practically?

- 100 grams of wholemeal bread: 60 grams of carbohydrate
- 100 grams of dry-weight pasta: 75 grams of carbohydrate
- 100 grams of beetroot/beets: 20 grams of carbohydrate
- 100 grams of mango: 20 grams of carbohydrate
- 1 banana: 25 grams of carbohydrate
- A 400-gram drained can of chickpeas: 39 grams of carbohydrate
- 200 millilitres of cow's milk: 10 grams of carbohydrate

WHAT DO WE MEAN BY CARBOHYDRATE AVAILABILITY?

Many people assume that carbohydrate availability is ensuring carbohydrate in the meal preceding exercise. We have already seen the importance of carbohydrate and the amounts required based on training load and intensity, so carbohydrate availability is ensuring sufficient carbohydrate is going to be available before, during and after training. Thus, depending on the training session, you may need to be thinking about this anywhere between twenty-four and seventy-two hours prior to your session.

So, if you were planning a moderate-intensity training session, with effort of around seven out of ten at 8 a.m. on Wednesday morning, you would need to think about your carbohydrate intake in the twenty-four hours prior to this.

An example (as a caveat, I want to say that this will depend on what training has occurred on Tuesday, and this is a basic guideline so you can see the types of food and frequency of eating to ensure carbohydrate availability. Amounts and volumes will vary from individual to individual):

Tuesday

- **Breakfast:** porridge made with milk, topped with walnuts and honey

- **Lunch:** beans on toast topped with cheese, and fruit and yoghurt smoothie

- **Mid-afternoon:** toasted tea cake or oat-based cereal bar

- **Evening meal:** pasta with roasted vegetables and chicken, followed by yoghurt and fruit

- **Before bed:** glass of milk and oatcake topped with peanut butter

Wednesday

In the morning, prior to the run, ensure that you take on a minimum of 30 grams of carbs which would be:

- Large banana

- 300-millilitre glass of juice

- Bagel (thin)

- Tea cake

- 1 Weetabix with milk

Within thirty minutes of completing your session, aim for 1 gram per kilogram of body weight of carbohydrate and 0.4 grams per kilogram of body weight of protein. This may be a drink such as a 300-millilitre carton of flavoured milk with a banana or a recovery shake, or it may be a second breakfast such as a toasted bagel with scrambled egg or granola and Greek yoghurt.

Protein

Proteins are the building blocks of the body, utilised widely for growth, maintenance and repair of muscle, as well as many other structures. Proteins are formed from chains of amino acids which, when broken down, are used in the production of DNA, red blood cells, hormones and enzymes, as well as for nutrient transport, immune response and cellular repair. Nine (or arguably eight) of the amino acids are essential for life and must be provided by the diet as they cannot be made within the body. These can be found as a complete source in animal products such as dairy, meat, fish and eggs, and as an incomplete source in plant-based proteins such as vegetables, grains, nuts and legumes. Plant-based proteins can be combined to provide the full range of essential amino acids. Some good combinations include baked beans on toast, rice and dhal, and a wholegrain bagel with peanut butter.

Athletes need protein primarily as a response to exercise rather than as a fuel source, although protein can be utilised for fuel when necessary and contributes towards 5–10% of daily energy requirements. During all exercise, including endurance sports, an increase in the breakdown of protein in the muscle has been shown to occur. Ensuring good protein choices, distributed throughout the day, helps to counteract these effects by aiding muscle protein synthesis – the rebuilding and repair of damaged muscle, as well as the building of new muscle. Taking on some protein soon after exercise may help to maximise recovery and training adaptation, but the post-exercise recovery window, once thought to be essential, is no longer considered as important as a regular intake of high-quality protein. Adequate protein intake is particularly important for older athletes in order to provide sufficient stimulus for muscle protein synthesis – this will be discussed in greater detail in chapter 8.

Protein requirements

A regular intake of high-quality protein is essential for repair, recovery and adaptation after exercise through muscle protein synthesis, as well as a source of fuel. Large amounts of protein ingested immediately after exercise aren't necessary, as most will simply be excreted by the body.

The recommended protein intake for endurance athletes is higher than for sedentary individuals by up to 1.2–1.4 grams per kilogram of body weight per day, ideally spread throughout the day, and for a 70-kilogram athlete equates to a little over 90 grams of protein per day.

The protein content of common foods is as follows:

- 100-gram portion of chicken or turkey breast: 30 grams of protein (an average chicken breast is 174 grams, which equals 52 grams of protein)
- 100-gram portion of oily fish or tinned tuna: 26 grams of protein
- 100 grams of red meat: 25 grams of protein
- 1 egg: 5 grams of protein
- 150 grams of Greek yoghurt: 15 grams of protein
- 100 grams of tofu: 8 grams of protein
- 200 millilitres of cow's milk: 7 grams of protein
- 200 millilitres of soya milk: 7 grams of protein
- 200 millilitres of almond milk: 1 gram of protein
- 100 grams of baked beans: 6 grams of protein (19.4 grams per can)

Fat

Dietary fat is essential for many biological processes. Apart from its role in providing energy, it has many important roles within the body, including for the formation of our cell membranes, for immune function, to absorb fat-soluble vitamins A, D, E and K, and to provide essential fatty acids that the body cannot make.

For many years, health messaging has focused on 'good' and 'bad' fats, suggesting we should all eat less saturated fats and more polyunsaturated fats for both our heart and our overall health. However, several recent high-quality studies are proving this approach is outdated and far too simplified, recommending instead that specific foods, rather than entire food groups, should be the focus of education and advice around dietary health.

A 2018 review found that different saturated fat types have different biologic effects and that including relatively high sources of saturated fats such as whole milk, dark chocolate and unprocessed meat in the diet does not raise the risk of cardiovascular disease (CVD). The authors concluded that 'there is no robust evidence that current population-wide arbitrary upper limits on saturated fat consumption [...] will prevent CVD or reduce mortality.'[5] Building on this research, a 2021 study in which the authors carried out not just novel research on 4,150 Swedish adults but also a review of past research, suggests that a higher intake of dairy fat is actually associated with lower CVD risk.[6]

So, while there is still much to be discovered about the role of different fats – and different sources of fat – in our diets, some messages at least are clear:

- Ultra-processed foods (which currently make up around 50% of the UK diet) and trans fats (hydrogenated or partially hydrogenated vegetable fats) are unequivocally linked to poorer health outcomes.
- Whole food sources of fats are likely to be the healthiest.
- Historical demonisation of fat and its replacement with carbohydrates (for example, in low-fat fruit yoghurts) is likely to have contributed to obesity and other negative health outcomes.
- Polyunsaturated fats include essential fatty acids and are considered beneficial to health. They include oily fish, such as salmon, sardines and mackerel, which are an exceptionally good source of omega-3 fatty acids; nuts and seeds, including their oils and butters; sunflower, rapeseed and olive oils; and avocados.

Fat requirements

A recommended 20–35% of daily energy intake should come from fat (around 1 gram per kilogram of body weight), with the majority coming from whole food sources:

- 25 grams of nut butter: 14 grams of fat
- 200 millilitres of whole milk: 7.4 grams of fat
- 100 grams of avocado: 15 grams of fat
- 20 millilitres of rapeseed oil: 18 grams of fat
- 25 grams of sunflower seeds: 13 grams of fat

- 100 grams of cheddar cheese: 30 grams of fat
- 1 mackerel fillet: 16 grams of fat

In certain situations, this recommendation of 1 gram per kilogram of body weight may need to be increased. Usually this will be linked to a training demand/adaptation or increased energy requirements. For example, athletes who train at high altitudes and cold temperatures, such as mountaineers and cross-country skiers, have huge energy demands while also contending with harsh conditions. For these athletes, increasing the overall percentage of energy from fat calories may be necessary.

Hydration

Staying hydrated is essential for optimal health. Add physical activity to this equation and it's even more important, as we will have more fluid losses to contend with in the form of sweat. Particularly in endurance sports, however, both under- and over-drinking can have serious consequences for health and performance.

Being dehydrated affects the body in many ways; most fundamentally it impairs the body's ability to regulate heat. During exercise, a rise in body temperature will lead to an elevated heart rate, and this in turn makes the perceived exertion at a given training intensity feel much harder and we fatigue more quickly. Additionally, mental function is reduced, leading to negative implications for decision-making, concentration and motor control. Another important symptom of dehydration is stomach discomfort; if we are dehydrated, any food we have consumed before or during training will stay in our stomach longer, potentially leading to gastric problems.

All the above factors will harm our exercise performance, meaning we won't get the best out of our training. However, the good news is that this can all be combatted if we learn to hydrate appropriately around our training, as well as on rest days. There are no specific guidelines for fluid intake because it depends on the type and level of exercise, and the environmental conditions, plus it also varies within individuals due to:

- genetics – some people innately sweat more than others
- body size – larger athletes tend to sweat more than smaller athletes
- fitness – fitter people sweat earlier in exercise and in larger volumes
- environment – sweat losses are higher in hot, humid conditions
- exercise intensity – sweat losses increase as intensity increases.

So how can we make sure we are getting enough fluid? The simple answer is by checking our urine colour. The ideal is that it is the colour of pale straw at all times. If it seems darker, especially before a training session, then drink. Get into the habit of monitoring thirst levels and drink throughout the day. One common mistake a lot of people make is that they don't drink enough through the day and then end up overloading their system prior to a training session.

When should we be eating?

Nutrient timing is an important part of fuelling for optimal recovery and consistency in training. Ideally this would include eating something one to three hours prior to your training session. If it is a higher-intensity session – that is, where you know you will be working at an effort of eight out of ten – you may also want to include some easily digestible carbs in the thirty minutes prior to the session.

If training is the stimulus which you have correctly fuelled, recovery food is now needed to make sure that the body can convert this stimulus to gains.

Ideally, recovery should be within twenty to thirty minutes of completing the session. If this falls outside of a mealtime, then it is recommended that you take this on in a liquid form, with a mixture of fast-release carbohydrate and easily digestible protein. This is why milk and milk products have become popular as recovery choices. The combination of carbohydrate and protein in a form that is easy to digest means your muscles receive the building blocks they need to help them repair and recover quickly and efficiently before the next training session. This should then be followed by a fully balanced meal within two hours.

If your recovery falls directly at a mealtime, then this next meal can be your recovery choice.

Generally, we recommend between 1 and 1.2 grams of carbohydrate per kilogram of body weight and 0.4 grams of protein per kilogram of body weight, repeated throughout the day at two- to three-hourly intervals, especially after a particularly long or high-intensity training session.

Some good suggestions for recovery nutrition include:

- milkshakes
- fruit and yoghurt smoothies
- eggs on toast
- chicken stir fry with noodles
- three-bean chilli and rice
- fish pie.

Sports nutrition

These specialised products provide a practical source of nutrients when it is impractical to consume everyday foods, such as during training or racing, or immediately before or afterwards. They include:

- sports/energy drinks
- sports gels
- sports confectionery, such as chews, bars and beans
- liquid meal supplements
- protein powders
- electrolytes.

The gut microbiome

While still a relatively new area of nutrition, there is no doubt that an important – and fascinating – link exists between our gut microbiome and both our mental and physical health. What is clear is that the more diverse our gut flora, the better it is for our health.

Made up of trillions of bacteria, fungi and other microbes, the gut's microbiome is unique to each person and has a number of functions, ranging from its impact on immune health and mental health to the synthesis of nutrients from our diet.

The environment in the gut is an ecosystem that is constantly changing and evolving. There are numerous factors that can influence its content and stability, including individual physiology and genetics, lifestyle, exercise, dietary composition and antibiotic use.

Below are some top tips on taking care of your gut microbiome.

1. Diet

Our diet is integral to so many aspects of life, from providing us with sufficient energy to allow for all the biological processes that keep us alive, to supporting our adventures and physical activity preferences. A diet that is too narrow or too restrictive, both in its variety of food types and/or energy provision, will negatively affect the gut microbiome.

So what should we eat for optimal gut health? Several key nutrients and food types have been identified which result in the increased microbial diversity that is recommended.

A high-fibre diet rich in colourful fruits, vegetables, legumes and wholegrain is central to increasing the bacterial diversity in our gut. While our body can't digest a high-fibre diet, there are certain bacteria in our gut that can, and this stimulates their growth, resulting in an improved environment.

Another food group that can be beneficial to include is fermented foods. These include yoghurt, sauerkraut, kombucha, kefir and tempeh. It has been found that including more of these foods enhances the function of the microbiome by reducing the abundance of disease-causing bacteria in the intestines.

A final word about diet: more research is needed, but it is something that should not be overlooked. Genetics plays a part in our microbiome, and to an extent the diets we have traditionally been brought up with in our families are most likely the ones that are going to ensure a more diverse and optimal microbiome for us as individuals. Thus, care needs to be taken when altering diets significantly. We know that not taking in sufficient food can result in dysbiosis – that is, changes to the microbiome – but, equally, if you have always had a mixed diet and suddenly change to becoming plant-based, it may take months or years before your gut adapts to this – if it ever does. Moving too far away from what your body has grown up with, while it may align with popular science, may not align with the body's overall health and performance.

2. Exercise

We know there are many benefits to being more physically active, but this does not necessarily mean everyone has to take up extreme challenges and high-intensity workouts. In fact, when it comes to our gut biome, any regular exercise of at least moderate intensity helps to decrease transient stool time (transit from the stomach through the colon), which offers protective properties against some diseases.

The key is ensuring some regular moderate activity through the week with good nutritional choices that not only support your training but also your gut health.

3. Probiotics

Probiotics are live micro-organisms, usually bacteria, that provide a specific health benefit when consumed. They work on the principle of colonising the gut, and benefit health by changing the overall composition of the microbiome and supporting metabolism. While they can be consumed daily, probiotics have been found to be most effective in restoring the microbiome to a healthy state after it has been compromised.

Care needs to be taken when using probiotic supplements, as most are destroyed by stomach acid and so don't make it as far as the gut. If you use a supplement, studies show those that are suspended in water can pass through the stomach unaffected.

Choosing a diet higher in fermented foods and live yoghurt will naturally boost probiotics, while including sufficient fibre will boost prebiotics which probiotics feed on.

When things go wrong: relative energy deficiency in sport (RED-S) and micronutrient deficiencies

Low energy availability and RED-S

Once thought to be an issue associated only with elite-level athletes, the prevalence of relative energy deficiency in sport (RED-S) is rapidly becoming better known in the wider fitness world, with recent figures suggesting that as many as 43% of recreational athletes, both male and female, are at risk of low energy availability.

Many of us strive to be the best we can at our chosen sport, navigating the daily stresses of work and family life at the same time, leaving us susceptible to being drawn in by promises of the latest fads and quick fixes. Surrounded by images of idealised body types presented through both mainstream and social media, and celebrities and influencers sharing the minutiae of their diets each day, it's easy to see how so many recreational athletes get lost along the way.

What do we mean by RED-S?

RED-S was previously known as the Female Athlete Triad, a combination of low energy availability, loss of menstruation and poor bone health. But this definition overlooked many of the complexities of the condition, as well as how low energy availability may present in male athletes.

RED-S occurs when there is not sufficient energy available for basic biological processes once the energy required for physical activity has been expended. When this happens, the ability to continue being physically active is prioritised, while some essential biological functions are reduced or cease altogether, with potentially damaging consequences for areas such as reproductive function and bone health, as well as athletic performance.

RED-S can either be intentional or unintentional

Unintentional or accidental RED-S occurs when an individual doesn't appreciate just how much energy is required to maintain both biological

41

function and training load. While they may present with similar symptoms to someone with intentional RED-S, rectifying the condition is usually much easier, as these individuals are happy to implement nutritional and training interventions to restore to optimal functioning.

Intentional RED-S results from a conscious decision to restrict energy intake and/or overtrain. Typically, it will involve some psychological aspects, including disordered eating behaviours and/or exercise dependency. Individuals often attribute the start of these behaviours to the desire to change their body composition, in most cases in order to lose weight. This may be because they have been encouraged to do so by the culture within their sport, through comparison to fellow athletes or through a belief that it will improve their performance.

Many athletes, particularly those who compete at a higher level, exhibit a specific set of personality traits. They may be driven, obsessive, focused, self-critical and perfectionist. While these exact traits are what make them good at their sport, if they are not managed appropriately, they can also be risk factors for dysfunctional behaviours, specifically around food, body image and training.

What happens in RED-S?

Our bodies have evolved to survive when conditions are lean, so, under conditions of chronic low energy availability, will down-regulate metabolism to preserve energy. Energy is taken away from repair and maintenance of internal systems, and also from reproductive function – having babies when food is scarce is clearly a bad idea.

Contrary to popular belief, RED-S is not always associated with a low weight or weight loss, and affected individuals – particularly those with a high percentage of lean mass – can present at normal or above-normal weight.

SIGNS AND SYMPTOMS OF RED-S

Physiological

- Cessation of periods, or a change to a previously regular menstrual cycle
- Decline in morning erectile function in male athletes (below five a week is a cause for concern)
- Changes to thermoregulation, difficulties staying warm in the winter and cool in the summer months
- IBS-like symptoms due to gastroparesis (slow movement of food through the digestive system) and dysbiosis (a change in optimal microbiome)

Performance

- Poor recovery between training sessions
- Recurrent injuries, including soft tissue, tendon and stress fractures
- Poor development of muscle mass and adaptation to training
- Increased risk and prevalence of infections and illness, making it difficult to train consistently

While the physiological and performance consequences are applicable to both types of RED-S, the following symptoms are mainly associated with those who have intentional RED-S.

Psychological/Behavioural

- Preoccupation and constantly talking about food
- Poor sleep patterns
- Restricting or strict control of food intake
- Overtraining or difficulties taking rest days
- Irrational behaviour
- Fear of food and weight restoration
- Severe anxiety
- Becoming withdrawn and reclusive
- An inability to decipher the difference between fact and intrusive thoughts and limiting beliefs

Diagnosis and treatment

RED-S is diagnosed by clinical assessment, including blood tests to rule out underlying conditions. Ideally, any individual who is identified as having RED-S should work with qualified clinical practitioners who have been trained in this speciality and who will also work collaboratively with medics, coaches and physios.

While a reduction in training is invariably required, it is not always necessary to stop all training when recovering from RED-S. This would only be encouraged if there was a serious risk to the individual's health or they were at a heightened risk of injury due to severe impact of their RED-S on their bone health. In most cases, manipulation and periodisation of training is suggested; this often means reducing intensity of training and encouraging some resistance training. The progression of this is dependent on physical, nutritional and clinical assessment, which will be determined by the treatment team.

Micronutrient deficiencies

I am an advocate of food first as a nutritional approach. I believe that, with a few exceptions, if you consume a balanced diet with sufficient energy to meet your requirements, then you should be able to also meet all your micronutrient needs. That said, there are some circumstances where you may need to consider supplementing your nutritional intake.

This might be due to juggling a high training load with a busy lifestyle, so recovery options need to be on-the-go, in the form of something like a shake. Perhaps you are going through a particularly high training load, making it difficult to meet the high demands through your diet alone. Again, in these instances, recovery drinks and high-energy snacks can ensure that you meet your requirements without adding too much bulk to the diet.

Additionally, female athletes who have heavy monthly menstrual bleeds may find that they need to supplement their diet with additional iron due to the high losses. Similarly, vegetarians and vegans will have certain vitamins and minerals that may be more difficult to absorb from a plant-based diet and thus will need to supplement.

With all this said, I have picked out some of the most common supplements that have a place and have been proven to be useful.

Iron

Iron is needed to make haemoglobin, which is the protein that transfers oxygen around the body. If iron levels become low, either due to a lack of intake or through excessive losses, this can manifest as iron-deficiency anaemia.

An inadequate intake of iron is possible if you are following a restricted diet for weight loss, and it is also often seen in athletes who may be suffering from RED-S. There is also a higher risk of deficiency if you are a vegan or vegetarian. Additionally, excessive losses can happen during menstruation in female athletes, but have also been linked to an increased breakdown in red blood cells in some runners particularly, due to the impact of the sport.

Why is iron deficiency such a big deal?

Iron is used to make haemoglobin – the oxygen-carrying part of our red blood cells. Without sufficient haemoglobin, the blood is able to transport less oxygen and must also work harder to deliver oxygen to where it is needed. This will not only make you feel pretty lousy, but will also have an impact on your overall performance.

Common symptoms to look out for include:

- feeling tired all the time
- being short of breath, even just going up the stairs
- poor performance in training
- dizziness
- looking pale
- loss of appetite
- bluish-tinted dark circles around the eyes.

If you have any of these symptoms, it would be worth going to talk this through with your GP, who can do a simple blood test to check your iron levels. Too much iron can be toxic, so don't be tempted to self-diagnose and start supplementing with iron without medical advice.

For vegetarians and vegans, who are at a slightly higher risk of iron deficiency than those who eat meat, combining vitamin C with plant-based iron-rich foods aids the absorption of iron, while drinking caffeinated beverages with meals inhibits absorption.

Iron-rich foods include:

- red meat
- fortified cereals
- dark leafy vegetables, such as spinach, kale and broccoli
- lentils and other pulses
- egg yolks.

ADDITIONAL FACTS

- There is no benefit (and potential harm) to taking an iron supplement if you do not have a deficiency of ferritin levels (iron stores) of less than 40 micrograms per litre.

- Low levels of both haemoglobin and ferritin reduce the ability to adapt to altitude.

- Low ferritin stores may increase the risk of stress fractures in those who are highly active.

Vitamin D

Along with several other important roles, vitamin D regulates calcium and phosphate in the body and is therefore essential for bone and muscle health. In the northern hemisphere, 80–90% of our required vitamin D is derived from skin exposure to ultraviolet B (UVB) radiation from sunlight, with the remaining 10–20% coming from our diets, from sources such as oily fish and fortified products. Particularly between September and April, this is the vitamin that people living in the UK are most likely to need to supplement. Those who spend a lot of time indoors, have darker skin pigmentation or cover their skin when outdoors, all of which reduce the absorption of UVB rays, may need to supplement all year round, along with older people, children and those who are pregnant or breastfeeding.

Symptoms of low vitamin D include:

- extreme fatigue
- muscle and bone pain
- low mood
- poor recovery between training sessions
- increased incidence of upper respiratory illness
- osteoporosis and increased risk of bone injury.

N-3 fatty acids

Also known as omega-3, these essential fatty acids play an important role in growth and development in children and young people. While there are many claims about their effectiveness in various areas of health, most research findings are inconclusive, although positive effects have been found for depression. The n-3 fatty acids eicosapentaenoic acid (EPA) and docosahexaenoic acid (DHA) are found in oily fish (derived from ingested seaweed), grass-fed meat, and eggs from chickens fed on a natural diet of insects and greens.

The n-3 fatty acid alpha linoleic acid (ALA) is found in foods such as walnuts, flax/linseeds and chia. Studies have shown that consuming these in your diet converts to a small amount of EPA. Similarly micro-algae oil supplements have shown to increase blood levels of both EPA and DHA but, to date, the dosage required is unknown.

It is recommended that athletes eat one or two servings a week to help meet their requirements. For those who are unable to hit this target, maybe due to palatability or dietary choice, a supplement may be advised.

B12

Vitamin B12, or cobalamin, is crucial to the normal function of the brain and the nervous system. It is also involved in the formation of red blood cells and helps to create and regulate DNA. The metabolism of every cell in the body depends on vitamin B12, as it plays a part in the synthesis of fatty acids and energy production. Vitamin B12 enables the release of energy by helping the human body absorb folic acid.

Chronic B12 deficiency affects the structure of blood cells, resulting in anaemia and, in some cases, nerve damage. B12 is not found in plant-based foods, so consuming fortified foods and supplementation is recommended for those following a plant-based or vegan diet.

Food supplements

According to the Food Standards Agency, a food supplement is defined as:

> 'any food the purpose of which is to supplement the normal diet and which is a concentrated source of a vitamin or mineral or other substance with a nutritional or physiological effect, alone or in combination and is sold in dose form'.[7]

The main aim of supplements aimed specifically at athletes is their ergogenic properties – those that have the potential to enhance performance. With numerous options and brands on the market, from sports drinks, gels, chews and recovery shakes to more specific individual nutrients such as caffeine, collagen and CherryActive, how do you know what works, what doesn't and when to take them?

When you are considering the use of a supplement, it is important to consider the balance between its potential benefits – is there evidence that this product will actually boost my performance? – and also the potential risks – is this product safe to use and is it stopping me from making better food choices?

The weight factor

'Lighter makes you faster' has traditionally been associated with endurance sports such as marathon running, triathlon and cycling. Similarly, being a lighter weight is necessary for weight-category sports such as lightweight rowing and martial arts, and power-to-weight ratio is important for climbing.

When we deep-dive into the research, there seems to be a direct correlation between additional weight and reduced running speed, but the key word here is 'additional' and so the benefits of a decrease in weight are generally associated with those individuals who start off at a higher weight and body-fat percentage than optimal for both health and performance. However, when it comes to getting lighter, there is a limit beyond which both health and performance start to decline. But what is that limit?

The difficulty is that the precise numbers are different for everyone, determined mostly by genetics, and the optimal weight and body composition for different sports also varies. For example, long-distance swimmers actually benefit from slightly higher body-fat percentages and mass.

Similarly, while BMI is not always ideal, as it doesn't take into account body composition, an optimal BMI for male 800-metre runners sits at 20–21, but drops to 19–20 in male 10,000-metre and marathon runners, which is most likely linked to the development of larger, heavier muscles in sprinters and middle-distance runners compared with endurance runners.

So it is clear that performance outcome is multi-factorial, and yet in certain sports the focus on a weight has a direct effect on participants' dietary behaviours. A study in *Frontiers* in 2019 looked at the dietary intake and eating attitude of recreational adolescent rock climbers.[8] The data showed that, with the exception of protein, this population group failed to meet their overall dietary targets for energy, fat and carbohydrate. The study did stress that, even with these results, they showed minimal risk of disordered eating, although this was still a concern within the climbing population. The study showed that 86% of climbers failed to meet their carbohydrate requirements, set at 5 grams per kilogram of body weight. These findings correlate with those in adult elite-level climbers, where 40% fail to meet their nutritional requirements. While this may not directly be related to disordered eating, it does demonstrate how certain beliefs around body size influence how an athlete eats and can often lead to accidental low energy availability or RED-S. Whether it is accidental or a conscious choice, low energy availability has negative consequences for both health and performance, as we described earlier.

Can you ever lose weight sensibly?

While the focus above has been on situations that can occur when losing weight is not necessary and becomes dysfunctional, as stated at the start of this chapter, we cannot ignore the fact that a very high percentage of the UK population is overweight and/or obese. Therefore, in certain cases, it will be legitimate to lose weight in order to improve health metrics.

We have seen that in some population groups, when an individual is heavier than is appropriate, losing weight can not only improve health but also improve performance. Thus, choosing methods that can help us to lose weight in a sensible manner can be of huge benefit.

Indeed, research shows us that when we focus on weight alone, we generally set people up to fail; but when the outcome results in reducing risk of heart disease, type 2 diabetes and blood pressure, it tends to encourage a change in behaviour.

We have seen that big deficits do not work. They just encourage the body to switch on compensatory behaviours, leading to weight regain. And yet, this is still the procedure that is advertised and encouraged: 'calories in' versus 'calories out'. It sets the scene and creates the belief that our bodies work in arbitrary units, rather than being a series of integrated processes that need constant attention.

The best way to lose weight, if it is necessary, is to consider behaviour change but also to make small changes daily. This not only leads to sustainable weight loss but ensures that what is lost is body fat and not muscle. When we encourage large deficits, and rapid immediate weight loss, we lose a lot of muscle too, which, along with the body's compensatory mechanisms, lowers our metabolic rate, as lean muscle mass burns more energy even at rest than fat.

Indeed, one thing to highlight relates to low-carbohydrate, high-fat (LCHF) diets. Many people who follow this approach report rapid immediate weight loss and see this as success. However, it is important to appreciate that this initial weight loss is just a loss of glycogen stores. Remember that carbohydrate is stored in our muscles as glycogen. For every gram of glycogen stored, we tend to hold 1–4 grams of water. This is not real weight loss, just a loss of water, and not related to a reduction in fat mass. It is also why when individuals reintroduce carbohydrate into their diets, they notice an immediate change to their weight, but once again, it is just stores being filled.

Weight loss is complex and involves both our physiology and psychology. What works for one person is not necessarily going to work for another. The key is choosing a process that is sustainable and achievable, but that is also not going to shut down your body. Making more nutrient-dense choices, ensuring sufficient carbohydrate around key sessions and slightly increasing your protein intake are all tried-and-tested methods that work well in athletes. The slightly higher protein intake not only preserves lean muscle mass losses when an individual is in a slight energy deficit, but also helps with satiety. Choosing to slightly increase your training while maintaining your present energy intake is best practice, as the body is biologically biased to achieve energy balance, and so we naturally increase our nutritional intake as we increase our training. Similarly if you try to do both together – that is, to increase training and reduce energy intake – you will create too big a deficit and your body will fight back. Remember, the science says no more than a loss of 100 calories a day results in the best outcome.

CHAPTER 2

Athlete Diets

Why do people – and specifically athletes – choose one diet over another?

Food consumption and behaviour are important yet complex topics, and often difficult to research accurately. Yet we know that in England 28% of the adult population are obese and a further 36% are overweight.[9] On the flip side of this, 16% of the adult population are known to have disordered eating or eating disorders, including binge eating.[10] While many lifestyle factors contribute to all the above situations, understanding what influences food choice or food avoidance is critical if we are to reduce all the above percentages.

According to statista.com, 34% of the UK population follow some set of nutrition rules, including 6% gluten-free, 6% lactose-free, 11% low-carbohydrate, 7% vegetarian, 5% pescatarian and 3% vegan.[11] The National Diet and Nutrition Survey's most recent results have demonstrated some significant changes, including a population decrease in the consumption of red meat, sugar and salt.[12] Comparatively, as a nation, we are still not hitting the recommended guidelines for fruit and vegetables. When we look at the key drivers that influence how we eat in the UK, there are myriad diverse factors, none of which are fully understood or predictable. However, the main considerations the UK population make are linked to:

- cost and perceived value for money
- availability and convenience
- marketing
- food safety
- food system actors, which include media, family, friends and academic environments
- clear and simple information.

When it comes to specific food choice, socio-economic status is a huge contributor, as well as the factors we discussed in chapter 1.

If we turn our attention to athletes, in those few studies and surveys that have been conducted, as one would expect, there appear to be factors specific to athletes that are particularly related to performance.

From the studies that have been done, the key factors that influence food choice in athletes are related to:

- performance
- food and health awareness
- weight control
- emotional influence
- influence of others
- food values and beliefs
- financial availability
- gut comfort.

An important finding is that, even with sufficient information, athletes don't always choose appropriate diets, with food preference and emotional influences rating highly among the key drivers of this.

What do athletes eat?

When it came to writing this book, I wanted to get an understanding of what food trends and approaches are most popular and why. The lack of existing data specific to athletes meant that I needed to do my own preliminary research, using a survey that asked questions to help me identify the most common diets being consumed. I reached out to a mix of male and female athletes from a range of different sports, backgrounds, competitive levels and adult age groups to ensure that the responses were as representative as possible. Participants were aware that this was research for a new book I was writing, but they had no further details about the topic of the book. So, while attempts were made to keep it neutral, we have to assume an aspect of bias, based on what athletes know about me, my knowledge and my experience.

SURVEY QUESTIONS

1. What sport do you participate in?

2. At what level do you compete/participate?

3. How many hours a week do you train?

4. Do you follow any specific dietary plan? E.g. plant-based, keto.

5. If yes, what influenced your decision to follow this method of eating?

6. How long have you been following this method of eating?

7. What potential benefits or problems have you encountered while following this plan?

8. If you are not following a specific way of eating, have you ever and if so what? Why? And why no longer?

9. Any other information about your nutrition and performance.

Although this was by no means a formal scientific study, and was a relatively small sample, the results were fascinating and the athletes demonstrated very similar trends and stated reasons for specific nutritional approaches.

There were clear correlations within sports, differences between sexes and nutritional strategies linked with sports performance. The following results were all based on the information that was collected through the survey, and no additional clinical observations were included.

From the 82 surveys that were sent out, 27 responses were from females and 55 from males.

The trends were as follows:

- The main reason given for changing diet was for performance benefits.
- The majority decided on their nutritional approach through reading an article or observing trends by other athletes on social media.
- Climbers were more likely to follow a low-carbohydrate, high-fat diet.
- Cyclists' preferences leant towards fasting, and particularly intermittent fasting.
- Runners were more likely to favour plant-based diets.
- While a previous diagnosis of RED-S was identified in all sports within the survey population, runners had the highest numbers, with female athletes being the higher percentage.
- Postmenopausal women were more likely to try low-carbohydrate, high-fat diets.
- 18% of the survey population had tried a low-carbohydrate approach to improve performance, but less than 1% had maintained this way of eating due to developing and then being diagnosed with RED-S, extreme fatigue or experiencing increased injury rates.

Informed by the responses from this survey, and the current popular dietary trends, chapters 3 to 6 look into each of the most popular approaches taken by athletes in greater detail, to help you make informed choices about the best diet to support your health and sport.

CHAPTER 3

Low-Carbohydrate Diets

The concept

In chapter 1 we discussed the role of carbohydrate in fuelling the body and brain. Stored as glycogen in our liver and muscles, we have between 1,600 and 2,000 calories – up to 120 minutes' worth – of carbohydrate-derived energy to call upon during exercise. While we are constantly burning both fat and carbohydrate, the higher the intensity of exercise, the more our bodies rely on our carbohydrate stores as an easily accessed source of energy, and the quicker it runs out.

In contrast, we have a huge store of energy that is relatively untapped, in the form of body fat – over 50,000 calories' worth for an average-sized athlete. Research has demonstrated that, through diet and training, our bodies can become more 'fat-adapted' – that is, better at prioritising fat as fuel. What if we could use this to our advantage, utilising more fat for fuel and sparing our precious carbohydrate stores, which could be advantageous especially in endurance events where high-intensity efforts are rare?

Low-carbohydrate, high-fat (LCHF) diets have become popular in recent years, both in athletic and non-athletic populations. Research has seen favourable results in people with high body-fat mass, insulin resistance or type 2 diabetes, but the picture for physically active people of healthy weight is much less clear.

What does it involve?

High-carbohydrate, low-fat (HCLF) diets, of the kind traditionally followed by endurance athletes, typically involve a carbohydrate intake of at least 45–65% of total daily calories (about 5 to 12 grams per kilogram of body weight per day) and a fat intake of 20–35% of total daily calories.

Conversely, low-carbohydrate, high-fat (LCHF) diets reduce carbohydrate intake to less than 25% of total daily calories, and increase fat intake to at least 60% of total daily calories. In practice, there is a wide range of both carbohydrate and fat values across individual approaches, even in those who claim to be on the same diet.

Most people lose weight rapidly when they first adopt a LCHF diet, but the majority of this weight loss will be due to the water that is stored alongside glycogen in the body, in a ratio of three parts water to one part glycogen. In weight-category sports such as boxing, rowing and martial arts, this rapid weight-loss aspect of a low-carbohydrate approach has been used for years to dip under a specific weight limit. But how does this stack up when it comes to both long-term health and athletic performance?

Pros and cons

There is no doubt that, in recent years, LCHF diets have gained momentum and a large and vocal following, both within athletes and the wider population. For overweight people who would legitimately benefit from a reduction in fat mass, and in particular those with insulin resistance – a precursor to type 2 diabetes, characterised by an impaired response to raised blood sugar that over longer periods of time can have massive detrimental effects on health – a low-carbohydrate diet may be helpful.

But it may not be the right choice for everyone, and there are convincing arguments against its efficacy for athletes.

One of the main arguments for the use and potential benefits of an LCHF diet in endurance and ultra-endurance events where performance is rarely at high intensity is that the body will become 'fat-adapted', leading it to prioritise using our abundant fat stores for fuel and sparing our much more limited glycogen stores. But there is a big downside to this. Becoming fat-adapted does make us better at utilising fat for fuel, but it also makes us worse at utilising carbohydrates. As well as affecting our ability to access readily available fuel provided by carbohydrates for shorter, more intense efforts, a LCHF diet significantly reduces the ability to use carbohydrate as fuel in any circumstance. This has the result of decreasing our metabolic flexibility – where we can quickly and easily switch between fuel sources depending on the body's requirements – and therefore our economy.

What do we mean by economy?

Economy is often used as a measure, particularly in endurance sports, and it measures the amount of oxygen used at a given speed. Good economy allows us to perform at a higher percentage of our maximum for longer, which is particularly important for events such as time trialling in cycling and marathon running. Specific training is the best way to improve economy but, interestingly, recent research demonstrated that while a LCHF diet improved fat oxidation in athletes, it also reduced economy, which, for those sports where the best economy determines who wins and who loses, is a serious problem.[13]

Even for ultrarunners, for whom long, slow, fat-fuelled running might make up a significant proportion of both training and racing, higher-intensity interval sessions, climbing hills and other necessary shorter, harder bursts of activity are still significant. Carbohydrate-based fuelling on the go during longer events also delivers rapid energy to muscles and the brain, and may be far more palatable and more easily digested than higher fat or protein options. So what's the best practical approach?

The most recent research explores the idea of periodising carbohydrate intake, by varying intake to match training and competition demands, but doesn't support an overall low-carbohydrate intake for athletic populations.[14] Indeed, there are more studies that demonstrate the pitfalls of a LCHF approach from both a health and performance point of view.

Periodising your carbohydrate around your training sessions is most definitely not about lowering or removing carbohydrate from your diet, but about choosing the most appropriate type of fuel for your activity type and level.

'Training low' means that you choose to do longer, slower or recovery sessions in a carbohydrate-depleted or fasted state. However, your carbohydrate requirements still need to be met through the rest of the day if optimal adaptation and progression is to occur.

Any benefits of training low must be balanced against an individual's risk factors. Those at risk of low energy availability, with high levels of stress aside from training, or who will struggle to refuel and recover sufficiently after training, should probably err on the side of caution and take on some carbohydrates before training. Either way, fasted or depleted training sessions should not be done more than twice a week and these should be undertaken at no higher than a perceived effort of six out of ten. Doing regular and/or high-intensity fasted sessions significantly increases the risk of illness, injury and underperformance and is, overall, more likely to be detrimental rather than beneficial.

Will an LCHF diet help me lose weight?

While many athletes choose the LCHF approach for performance, there are some who see it as a way of losing weight and achieving a weight target.

As always, the scientific findings are mixed, with some studies supporting this method of weight loss and others not doing so. Many of the studies that support following LCHF diets for weight loss are short-term (three to six months), and also in the general population, not the athletic, with no follow-up beyond twenty-four months, and thus long-term adherence or outcomes are unknown.

Aside from the initial loss of water weight, one of the main reasons often stated as to why a LCHF diet can support weight loss is that fat and protein have a higher satiety value – that is, they stop us feeling hungry more quickly, reducing the risk of overeating. However, while this would make sense due to the higher energy yield of fat, and the slower digestion time of both fat and protein compared with carbohydrate, the fact remains that it is the overall energy balance that has the greatest effect on body weight, regardless of the source of that energy. A 2021 study that looked at the effect of a plant-based, low-fat diet versus an animal-based, ketogenic diet on the participants' daily, unrestricted energy intake demonstrated some interesting findings.[15] In this study, subjects were randomly assigned to either a low-fat, plant-based diet which provided 78% energy from carbohydrate and 10% energy from fat, or a LCHF diet which provided 78% from fat and 10% from carbohydrate, for a two-week period. After this period, both groups swapped to the other nutritional approach for a further two weeks.

The results showed that when the subjects were on the low-fat, plant-based diet, their overall energy intake was significantly lower. On average they consumed around 600 fewer calories a day than when they were on the LCHF diet. In addition, it was noted that despite the lower energy intake during the low-fat, plant-based diet, the LCHF diet led to more rapid early weight loss during the first week, but total weight loss after two weeks was not significantly different. When body composition was investigated, it helped to explain these results; only the low-fat, plant-based diet resulted in significant loss of body fat, whereas the LCHF diet led to loss of fat-free mass – that is, muscle and fluid. The author of the study made it very clear that this research was to investigate different dietary approaches on *ad libitum* (unrestricted, chosen by the participants) energy intake and was not specifically looking at weight loss. It was also relatively short-term and didn't look at a 'normal' Western diet, which typically contains a lot of ultra-processed foods high in both simple carbohydrates and fats. However, what it does show us is that a LCHF diet is not always going to lead to helpful weight loss.

Case studies and discussion

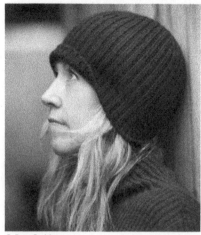

© Pete Stables

HOLLY'S STORY

I have known Holly for over ten years, first as a peer at our local running club, which developed into a great friendship, and subsequently I have been supporting her with nutrition advice for some of her key races, especially as she transitioned into the world of ultras.

I previously ran marathons and represented GB at the European Athletics Championships, 2010, and England at the Commonwealth Games, Delhi, 2010. Since then, I have also run for GB at numerous trail and mountain events, but I would consider myself ex-elite now, albeit still a very competitive runner.

From early on in my marathon career, I became quite fixated on achieving a particular race weight; while I didn't avoid any food groups at this stage, I can see now that I hugely under-fuelled for my training load. During this time I suffered with hypothalamic amenorrhoea due to low energy availability, and subsequently this resulted in numerous stress fractures and also my move away from road to trail.

In 2013 I decided to try the LCHF approach to 'fat-adapt'. This was also to support my move from road marathons to ultra-distance trail events. The first week was tough – I experienced brain fog and fatigue – but soon after I started to notice how great I felt. I had no stomach issues, and my energy levels were improving.

However, about six months down the line I started to notice real issues with fatigue once again, an inability to maintain pace in sessions, and my heart rate skyrocketed both at rest and while training. I went to see a sports doctor, who after numerous tests diagnosed EBV (Epstein–Barr Virus), because of the low-carbohydrate diet depressing my immune system.

It took many months for me to recover, which included reintroducing carbohydrate and significantly modifying my training. I was unable to compete for eighteen months. My periods did return sporadically but I was still very prone to injury.

Since then, I have changed my whole approach to training and diet. I now run up to 80 miles a week with very few double days, I strength-train two to three times a week and I eat everything. I no longer restrict my overall intake and I focus on ensuring carbohydrate availability, especially around my training sessions.

I am stronger and more resilient as an athlete; I no longer think about food all the time and have noticed that my body regulates. While my weight is not the ideal I had previously set myself, I am much leaner now than when I was restricting.

....

PROFESSIONAL OPINION

While Holly's dysfunctional relationship with food and her weight started a few years before, she paid the price when it came to a LCHF approach. One could argue that as a female she was at a higher risk of her body being sensitive, or that it was the volume of high-intensity load that still made up a significant percentage of her training, but, whatever the reason, it put her body and performance under a lot of strain. While the LCHF approach is advocated in endurance athletes, it is important to be mindful that there is little scientific backing, especially in those athletes who include a range of intensities in their training for maximum progression. While there may be a place for certain sessions to be done in a fasted or carbohydrate depletion, this doesn't translate as low- or zero-carbohydrate.

....

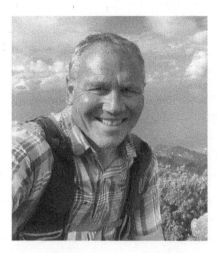

STEPHEN'S STORY

Stephen and I don't know each other as such, but he works at Vertebrate Publishing and was keen to discuss how his change to eating a high-fat, low-carbohydrate diet has impacted his life and performance.

I have always struggled to manage my weight and I started running because I thought that would help keep it under control. It seemed to work but, more importantly, I enjoyed running and then started entering races – half marathons and then marathons from the age of twenty-two onwards. My highlight was running the 1985 London Marathon, at the age of twenty-three, in just under three hours. At that time I weighed around 84 or 85 kilograms and that seemed about right for me. I have broad shoulders and a reasonably heavy frame.

As I got older, work and family made it harder to run as much and my weight bounced around and probably peaked at somewhere over 100 kilograms in my forties. I would run intermittently but it was often hard.

Fifteen years ago we moved and I could get out more. I ran a lot but was too heavy and struggled to lose weight. I tried all sorts of things, even giving up alcohol for seven years, but it was a constant battle and I had to run further and further to keep my weight stable.

I've always loved reading about running and have a shelf full of books, including *Lore of Running* by Tim Noakes, a pioneer in his work on hydration whilst running and the role of the brain in controlling physical performance. He was a keen runner and highly regarded sports scientist, and his book supported the generally accepted view that runners should eat lots of carbohydrates. At a similar age as I am now, Dr Noakes was battling against weight gain and running further and further to try and control it but not succeeding. He (re)discovered the low-carb, high-fat diet and it had a dramatic impact on his weight and health, such that he began proselytising about the diet. This led to professional complaints against him by the Health Professions Council of South Africa and he wrote up the resulting court case where his professionalism and also the efficacy of the diet were both vindicated.

So, I decided to do the same. One day I ran for two hours, then just decided I would eat no more carbs. I read lots of books and visited some fantastic websites and found that it was possible to stay in a ketogenic state, where the body burns its own fat as long as carbs are limited to 50 grams per day. This is about the amount in one piece of toast or a small banana, but I also found it is about the same as two bottles of beer. I had found that beer was good for stopping my legs twitching in the evening, so thought the perfect diet was no carbs and maybe a beer or two if I had run earlier that day. One difference I had to cope with, compared to the diet Tim Noakes advocates, is I don't eat meat. Fortunately, we keep hens, so that meant lots of eggs in addition to nuts, cheese and canned fish.

I started in June 2019 and I was reasonably fit, having just run the London Marathon with my kids in just over four hours. But I was 96 kilograms and my blood pressure was too high. I was starting a course of treatment and it seemed that I would have to be taking quite a few different types of pills to get it to an acceptable level. I have a history of high blood pressure, but have generally just ignored it.

On the second day into this new way of eating, I stopped feeling hungry. I realised that what I had thought was hunger was just a craving for carbohydrates and that soon went. Sometimes, I could go all day without eating or thinking about food.

Running was a different matter, and for the first couple of weeks I felt terrible. Worse than the last few miles of any marathon. My 10k daily runs went from taking fifty minutes to well over an hour.

My weight started to come down (settling at around 83 kilograms) and my body gradually became used to operating without carbs. I started running faster up the hills, but that was because I was carrying less weight.

I thought I was fully adapted after six to eight weeks, but then at three months I really started to feel a lot quicker and more energetic. I was beating times I had set over the last fifteen years, some when my weight had been at low levels. Age-graded tables would suggest I should have been 10–15% slower. My blood pressure came down and my cholesterol levels were also fine.

So, I felt better, I ran faster and my new diet seemed to suit my body. Then I realised there was another huge benefit – I was completely independent of food.

One of the difficulties of moving away from carbs is that it can be very hard to find suitable food. Virtually everything made in factories seems to contain sugar or starch in various combinations. At first this was a problem, but then I realised that if I wasn't hungry there was no reason to eat then and I could just use my body's stores of fat for fuel. I have completely lost any sense of ever needing food at a particular point in time.

Not needing to keep fuel topped up is a huge advantage when doing endurance events and has made them far more enjoyable. I started doing five- to six-hour runs in the mountains and took nothing other than a cup to drink from streams. Then I completed the OMM in October 2019 and ran two tough back-to-back days of seven and five hours with only a couple of stock cubes overnight. Every extra gram you carry on your back counts, so there is just no point in carrying food if you don't need it. When I finished, the only thing on offer was falafel wraps, which I decided were too high in carbs and just didn't need. I don't think I ate until I got home from Scotland on Sunday night.

In July this year I set off to do the 82-mile Dales Way with a rucksack containing, amongst other things, tent and sleeping bag and full camping equipment, as I planned on taking three days and maybe camping and eating in pubs along the way. I took no food other than some emergency jelly babies (I always take these in case I have some problem which I think sugar might solve, but have never needed them) and a bottle to collect water from streams along the way. I started in the middle of the day and was enjoying it so much and felt so good that I just carried on through the night and finished in the middle of the next day. I had no food and was never hungry.

In October I did something similar, running/walking 65 miles of the coast-to-coast route (3,500-metre climb) in around twenty-one hours, again with no food. My friend had to stop numerous times for resupply along the way, and also suffered stomach problems, which I never have.

So, for eighteen months I have not any eaten sweets, cakes, biscuits, potatoes, bread, pasta, below-the-ground vegetables, energy bars, bananas, apples – anything runners usually eat. Instead, I eat fish, nuts, green vegetables, dairy and the occasional piece of 90% chocolate. I still drink one or two beers each day, and run around 70 kilometres a week, all off-road and hilly. My friends and family think I am disciplined, but it really is easy as I just never crave any of those things.

....

PROFESSIONAL OPINION

I want to state as a caveat here that personally I never like to discuss actual numbers when mentioning weight. However, all the case studies have been written by the individual and so I didn't want to lose the essence of what they were trying to capture and discuss.

It is clear that Stephen's main priority was trying to lose some weight, but it is also clear in his case that this loss in mass was legitimate. While he has lost weight, he has returned to what feels like his 'set point weight', as this is where he sat naturally during his younger years and you could argue that it has been the change in lifestyle and being more mindful of nutrition that has actually caused this loss.

It is clear that this approach is working for Stephen; it has helped him to avoid energy slumps and sugar craving. Stephen has found a balance that seems to work for him, as he still includes a couple of beers, some dairy and carries jelly babies in case of emergencies, which would suggest that his economy has been impacted by his approach and so when changes in terrain result in a higher intensity, his body still looks to run on sugar. While Stephen covers a large volume of miles every week, it is possible that if these are all done at a relatively easy to steady pace, his body and performance is not affected by the lack of carbohydrate. Exercise alone doesn't necessarily lead to weight loss, especially as we get older. It is important to remember that our body does like to achieve energy balance, and usually if we increase our energy output through training, then we also increase our energy intake. It would be interesting to see if reducing his volume of training and increasing an element of resistance training would allow Stephen to maintain his present weight, while also improving his body composition and eating more carbohydrate, especially wholegrain, which would support gut health.

We know that no two humans are the same and so finding the approach that works for you is essential. That said, it is also relatively early into his journey with this way of eating and it is important that Stephen is aware of the potential impact this approach may have on his health and performance. We will also highlight in later chapters why this approach is less suitable for females.

Summary of key points

There is no doubt that the LCHF approach has become popular amongst athletes of all levels and abilities, although the controversy around its benefits both for health and performance is apparent.

The large range of studies available that have looked into the impact of LCHF diets makes it difficult to advocate this approach as a sports-nutrition professional, especially with more data highlighting the negative consequences, particularly to long-term health. However, we know that no two people are the same, and thus different approaches to training and nutrition need to be considered. Genetics, gender, lifestyle and training age all have a part to play.

CHAPTER 4

Vegan and Plant-Based Diets

The concept

As of 2021, 12% of the adult UK population were following a vegetarian (7%) or pescatarian (5%) diet, and 3% followed a vegan diet, with younger demographics making up by far the larger part in all cases. Plant-based diets are big business, too: the UK meat-substitute market is worth an estimated 500 million euros and growing.[16] Netflix documentaries like *The Game Changers*, the increased plant-based narrative on social media, and elite athletes from a wide range of sports advocating the switch for environmental, health and performance benefits, all add to the visibility of plant-based eating – in fact, it's impossible to ignore.

The term 'plant-based' can often be interchanged with both vegan and vegetarian diets, so how is it actually defined?

While all three terms avoid – to a greater or lesser extent – the consumption of animal-based products, there are some key differences. In general, when we use the term 'plant-based' we are inferring that the individual predominantly chooses to avoid consumption of animals and animal products due to health or environmental reasons. Like vegetarianism, eating a plant-based diet does not necessarily involve avoiding products or services that have the potential to cause suffering to animals. For instance, someone who eats a plant-based diet may choose to wear leather or use personal care products that contain animal-derived ingredients. Unlike strict vegetarians, though, being plant-based does not mean you always avoid meat or meat products; you may still include them in your diet on occasion.

Being vegan is a philosophy and a lifestyle choice. In fact, The Vegan Society use the following definition:

> Veganism is a philosophy and way of living which seeks to exclude – as far as is possible and practicable – all forms of exploitation of, and cruelty to, animals for food, clothing or any other purpose; and by extension, promotes the development and use of animal-free alternatives for the benefit of animals, humans and the environment. In dietary terms, it denotes the practice of dispensing with all products derived wholly or partly from animals. [17]

In comparison, being vegetarian involves eating a diet that excludes meat, fish and animal ingredients such as gelatine, but still includes eggs, dairy foods and honey. However, unlike plant-based, it is a dedicated practice, not one you occasionally consume.

The main distinction between a vegetarian diet and a vegan diet is that vegetarians avoid foods that involve killing animals, but do not avoid all animal products. Vegetarians see eating eggs and dairy foods as acceptable, whereas vegans argue that the practice constitutes cruelty and exploitation.

When we look at the science, there is a strong argument for eating a more plant-based diet for health, animal welfare and environmental reasons. Studies investigating optimal health and longevity of life are clear that a Mediterranean-style diet with a high intake of wholegrains, brightly coloured fruit and vegetables and essential fatty acids has positive links with improved quality of life and less prevalence of disease. Although a

Mediterranean diet is neither vegetarian nor vegan, it does demonstrate a good example of being plant-based, particularly in comparison to a traditional Western diet, as it contains a lot more fresh produce but foods from animal origin are still included, with some – such as oily fish – actively encouraged.

To date, there are no conclusive studies that show that a plant-based diet is necessarily superior to a mixed diet from a health perspective; but equally, if followed appropriately, it may contribute to some improved health metrics, such as a more balanced gut biome, lower susceptibility to heart and metabolic diseases, and healthier body composition; but as a necessary caveat, this is based on a well-balanced and fresh-ingredient approach to a plant-based diet.

While the statistics point to a huge rise in people following a plant-based diet, they also show a concurrent rise in demand for ultra-processed and takeaway options. Consideration of dietary choices is essential, regardless of the specific diet followed, and just because a product is labelled as vegetarian or vegan, it doesn't automatically mean it's healthy.

Diet choice is far from being just about health. Long before veganism and plant-based eating became on-trend and part of the emerging 'wellness world', many of those who adopted this approach did so due to the moral arguments around animal welfare. While this is still one of the key influences for following this way of eating, another important factor is the impact meat and dairy production has on the environment and climate change. In fact, some would argue that this is presently top of the leader board contributing to the huge rise in plant-based eating. As US academic and philosopher Gary L. Francione, who has written extensively on ethics around animal welfare and environmentalism, states:

> The bottom line is clear: we are facing imminent disaster. If we really want to save the planet from climate catastrophe, we must promote a grassroots effort with a clear normative directive: stop eating animal products and adopt a vegan diet. [18]

But it's surely too simplified to say 'vegan good, animal bad', as there are many vegan products, particularly those that are highly processed and packaged with unsustainable ingredients that are catastrophic in their contribution to climate change. To truly be as ethical as possible, a diet, regardless of its specific rules, should be one that prioritises food that is seasonal, and locally and organically produced where feasible. Is it better to drink organic milk produced and bought from your local farm or a plant milk made from heavily sprayed crops or almonds grown with high water usage in drought-prone areas? Or a product that substitutes butter for air-freighted palm oil from plantations that destroy vast swathes of biodiverse forest?

Plant-based diets and athletes

It is clear that the number of people adopting a plant-based diet is on the rise. Data on the athlete population is limited, with the most recent prevalence results available being from the 2010 Commonwealth Games, which reported 8% of the athletes following a vegetarian diet, of whom 1% were vegan.[19] However, if we follow the population trends, particularly when younger people are more likely to follow a plant-based diet, then we have to assume that this growth is also apparent in athletes. Indeed, the data from our survey would support this theory. While some of the athletes we spoke to had made the change for both animal welfare and environmental reasons, the majority chose this approach due to the potential perceived benefits to their performance.

Once again though, when sorting through the literature, there is a real lack in empirical data looking at the direct impact of vegan diets specifically on athletic performance. Studies do show that performance is unaffected in those athletes who choose a vegetarian diet, but the specific information on vegan diets is scant.

That said, in general, there is absolutely no reason why a vegan diet cannot support an athletic lifestyle if it is carefully constructed. The general sports nutrition guidelines around macronutrients and energy availability are just as applicable, regardless of the specifics of a diet.

Pros and cons

There is no denying that a well-balanced, nutrient-dense, plant-based diet can wholly support athletic performance. However, to date, and despite the claims by several high-profile athletes, there are no studies that prove that removing all animal products is superior from a performance point of view.

Anecdotally, it is possible that those athletes who have seen an improvement have simply improved the overall quality of their diet by making a change that requires them to be more considered and mindful about the choices they make, compared with a previous diet.

The case for eating more plant-based food with regard to improving our long-term health is well established, even if this is through a more flexitarian approach, with the focus on cooking with fresh ingredients from scratch whenever possible.

A plant-based diet is likely to make it easier for an athlete to hit their carbohydrate requirements and recommendations for fruit and vegetables, especially as they are likely to include a greater range of grains, pulses and fresh produce in order to meet their energy requirements. However, on the flip side of this, the typically high fibre content of a vegan diet and naturally low energy content of available foods may result in early satiety – feeling full – and could mean that, over time, the athlete fails to meet their energy requirements, leading to detrimental impacts on health and performance.

What about protein?

I'm often asked whether it's possible to meet the protein requirements of athletes, particularly older athletes, through a vegan diet.

In general, the role of protein is in the response to exercise, maintaining and repairing our bodies in the background, although it can also be used as fuel if necessary. Muscle protein synthesis is the process by which muscle is generated and repaired, encouraged both by protein intake and the exercise stimulus. Ensuring sufficient dietary protein, with intakes spaced out through the day, is the best way to promote optimal recovery and adaptation.

While there appears to be little significant difference between vegetarian and mixed diets with regard to protein intake, vegans may struggle to source sufficient high-quality protein, and in particular complete proteins, containing all nine essential amino acids. Special attention is needed not just around the quantity but also the quality of protein, combining sources to ensure that the full complement of amino acids is included.

One key essential branched-chain amino acid that has been shown to be significant in muscle protein synthesis is leucine; cow's milk seems to have a superior effect on muscle protein synthesis because of its high leucine composition. Plant-based milk options are generally low in protein concentration, due to how they are manufactured, but are devoid of leucine. Pulses such as lentils and peas are good plant sources of leucine, but at lower concentrations than in dairy.

One final point to consider is digestibility. This is important as it measures the uptake into the body and influences response to, and adaptation from, training. Animal protein sources tend to be more easily digestible, but taking in plant-based proteins in the form of nut or seed butters or powders helps to counteract this. Recent research has found that vegan athletes who supplement with plant protein powders seem to have like-for-like responses when compared with whey-based protein powders.

What's missing?

Micronutrients

With the exception of vitamin B12, a well-constructed plant-based diet along with adequate sunlight should be able to provide all required micronutrients. Vitamin B12, as discussed in chapter 1, is essential for many body processes, including brain and neurological function, and only occurs in very low levels in plants. The Vegan Society takes a firm line on B12:

> In over 60 years of vegan experimentation only B12 fortified foods and B12 supplements have proven themselves as reliable sources of B12, capable of supporting optimal health. It is very important that all vegans ensure they have an adequate intake of B12, from fortified foods or supplements.[20]

Vitamin D is also more difficult to get from a vegan diet, so those who may not be exposed to sufficient sunlight for vitamin D synthesis in the body should also consider taking a vitamin D supplement.

Iron

Iron deficiency is relatively common in the athletic population, particularly in female endurance athletes, probably due to a combination of menstruation and muscle breakdown. Anaemia can result, due to a reduction in the iron-dependent oxygen-carrying haemoglobin, leading to symptoms such as tiredness and fatigue, weakness, shortness of breath and reduced exercise tolerance. Iron deficiency *without* anaemia, which has been shown to be more prevalent in plant-based athletes, has also been found to reduce endurance capacity, increase energy expenditure and impair adaptation to endurance exercise in females.

One way around this is to consume iron-rich foods in the presence of foods high in vitamin C, to enhance the absorption of iron from plant-based sources.

Calcium

The body's calcium requirements are more difficult, though by no means impossible, to meet through a plant-based diet, particularly in vegans. A 2020 review of the literature showed that due to lower intakes of calcium, those who followed a plant-based diet were at a higher risk of fractures.[21]

Plant-based sources of calcium include nuts, soya, beans, green leafy vegetables and fortified foods. It's worth noting that some leafy vegetables, such as spinach, contain high levels of oxalates, which compromise absorption of calcium.

Iodine

Vegans in particular may be at risk of iodine deficiency, due to the low levels in plants and grains compared with animal-derived foods. Iodine has an extremely important role to play in thyroid function and metabolism. Iodine is abundant in seaweed, but care should be taken not to overcompensate by over-ingesting iodine. Where iodine requirements cannot be met through diet, and, crucially, a deficiency is medically diagnosed, supplementation may be required.

Case study and discussion

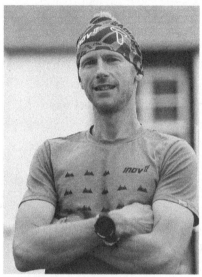
© inov-8.com/Dave MacFarlane

DAMIAN'S STORY

Damian and I met through running. We are both Bath-based and both authors. Damian contacted me around the time *Training Food* was published as he was about to embark on his first multistage ultra and wanted some nutritional tips. Since then, I have continued to provide him with advice as and when he has required it. Two years ago, Damian also became my coach.

I rediscovered the addictive joy of running as part of a tame midlife crisis, doing my first half marathon aged thirty-five. I soon ran my first marathon (dressed as a toilet – and, yes, I did look a bit flushed) and ultramarathon, and four years after that I was somehow in the GB team at the Trail World Championships. Setting records on Britain's National Trails and placing in the top ten at Ultra-Trail World Tour races, including the Ultra-Trail du Mont-Blanc, has led to sponsorship and other wonderful opportunities, including films and books. I've become a semi-professional athlete and full-time running coach. It's been life-changing. And has taught me that fourth breakfast is a real thing.

Like most people, I say I care about nature. But in 2019 the compelling Extinction Rebellion protests in London made me realise how urgent action is. I've become really worried about our climate and ecological emergency. Scientists say we must cut global CO_2 emissions by 45% this decade and it's just not happening anywhere near fast enough. System change will have so much more impact than individual changes. But I think they can help too, even if just by keeping the topic salient.

Avoiding meat and dairy is the 'single biggest way' to reduce your impact on Earth, concluded a 2018 study published in the journal *Science*.[22] Animals are ace (especially cats and squirrels), but I'd also enjoyed eating chicken while trying not to think too much about how it arrived on my plate. Red and processed meat also gets linked to some nasty diseases. So I had three strong reasons to give veganism a try.

It's been so much easier and more fun than I imagined. There's loads of tasty stuff around. I'm probably eating more healthily too. Renee, who's been advising me since almost day one of long-distance running, warned me I may need some supplements, and I take vitamin B12, D3 and a multivitamin. I do sometimes think back on my day and realise there wasn't much protein, but that's easily fixed with some pea protein powder or hummus on toast. And sometimes I'm hungry at 9 p.m. But again, that's easily fixed with nut butter on toast. Most things can be fixed with toast.

I don't know if it's affected my athletic performance either way. But a recent blood test result was the best I've had. Plus, I feel better ideologically because I'm behaving in accordance with a value. And that feels good.

....

PROFESSIONAL OPINION

Damian's story is a perfect example of how understanding the importance of fuelling for training and how to achieve your requirements on a plant-based diet can support performance while maintaining your personal moral values.

It is clear from the above account that Damian tunes into his body and knows when he needs to adjust his intake to ensure optimal intake. While we would hope this would be the case for all athletes, sadly there have been some accounts where a plant-based diet has been followed as a way of cutting out food groups. In these instances, chronic under-fuelling is a huge risk which can then lead to further health and performance consequences.

Summary of key points

When constructed carefully, plant-based, vegetarian and vegan diets can all, without doubt, support a healthy, low-impact lifestyle. When considering athletes specifically, care needs to be taken to ensure that overall energy, protein and key micronutrient requirements are met in order to support optimal performance and health. As with all nutritional approaches, some individuals will definitely respond better than others.

For those choosing a plant-based diet for ethical reasons – animal welfare and climate change being the primary reasons stated – food choices should be carefully considered. Heavily packaged or processed foods, or those containing ingredients such as unsustainably sourced palm oil and soya, which may have hugely negative indirect consequences to their production, should be avoided.

CHAPTER 5

Intermittent Fasting

The concept

Intermittent Fasting (IF) was first made popular in the general population as a means of weight loss by BBC journalist Michael Mosley with the broadcast of his 2012 documentary, *Eat Fast and Live Longer*. Since then, there have been numerous others who have followed in his footsteps.

There are two main versions of IF. The first one involves a prolonged period of fasting and a specific 'window' to consume food, with the best-known being 16:8, where the individual consumes their meals within an eight-hour window and fasts for sixteen hours. The timing is up to the individual, but it needs to be maintained. So, if they choose to eat between 12 p.m. and 8 p.m., then they would fast from 8 p.m. until 12 p.m. While this is the most popular approach, new variations have been introduced, such as 12:12 and 14:10.

The second approach is more complicated and involves a 5:2 pattern where you eat 'normally' on five days of the week and then, for the remaining two days, limit your intake to just 500 calories a day. Similarly to the time-restricted version of IF, different people follow different patterns, including alternate-day fasting. This involves eating as normal on alternate days and limiting intake to 500 calories on the other days.

Beyond the possibility of weight loss, proponents of IF diets suggest they can slow down the ageing process, reduce oxidative stress, improve the gut microbiome, improve body composition and improve metabolic biomarkers; but so far, longer-term studies haven't been conclusive on any of these outcomes.

Aside from its proposed health benefits, fasting is also undertaken for religious practice and beliefs. During the month of Ramadan, Muslim adults do not eat during daylight hours. Ramadan falls in the ninth month of the Islamic calendar, which changes yearly, based on the cycles of the moon. It marks the month the Qur'an, the Muslim holy book, was first revealed to the Prophet Muhammad. During Ramadan it is common for Muslims to consume one meal just before dawn, and a second directly after sunset.

So where does IF fit in with athletic performance?

From our survey, while it wasn't one of the most popular options, IF was mentioned on several occasions but, interestingly, only by cyclists. Much of the previous research around fasting in athletes has focused on fasting for religious reasons. However, a 2019 review of the literature around intermittent fasting in athletes concluded that, across 'high-intensity, endurance, and resistance exercises, studies have been varied but are uniform in showing that there is no benefit to athletic performance while fasting'.[23]

Pros and cons

While there does not appear to be a specific benefit to athletes from following an IF approach compared with any other calorie-restricted diet, there may be indirect benefits to athletes resulting from other effects.

A 2020 review of the literature concluded that IF may be effective in reducing obesity, improving body composition, reducing insulin resistance and controlling blood pressure in some people – but only as effective as more traditional calorie-controlled diets.[24] Unlike simple calorie restriction, however, which is notoriously difficult to adhere to, IF may be easier to plan and follow, with no particular food groups being restricted or avoided altogether. Indeed, the athlete can eat *ad libitum* – that is, how they want to – with the key being that intake needs to be restricted to the eight-hour window. But this fact alone makes it even more important to emphasise the message that there is no substitute for a nutrient-dense and varied diet, based mostly on plants and with minimal processed foods.

In some cases, IF may interfere with the timing of training and fuelling/refuelling around training. For those with no alternative but to train in the early mornings or evenings, for example, it may be difficult to fit in training during non-fasting times, with the consequence that either the quality of training or recovery may be negatively affected. Similarly, if following the 5:2 plan, training will need to be scheduled on days when fuelling is sufficient to cover both training and metabolic processes.

Performance-wise, it is clear from the research available that there don't appear to be any direct benefits of intermittent fasting for athletes, although there is the potential for its indirect effects to positively affect health and performance. However, for many athletes, particularly those already at risk of low energy availability, one could argue that training in a depleted/fasted state not only impacts performance but, as we saw with LCHF diets, can impair recovery and depress the immune system, increasing the risk of injury, infections and illness.

Case studies and discussion

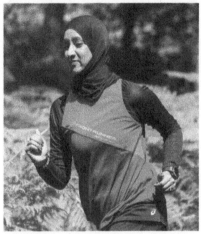
© Tanya Raab

TAZ'S STORY

Taz and I have been ambassadors for a couple of different running brands at the same time. During this time, I have enjoyed getting to know Taz but have also been inspired by how she has been challenging cultural beliefs and really flying the flag for Asian women and running.

In Islam, there are five key practices or pillars that all Muslims are obligated to fulfil throughout their lifetime, and fasting in Ramadan is one of them – i.e. it is an act of worship. Muslims follow the lunar calendar and therefore the start and end date is usually a prediction. Because the lunar year is ten days shorter than the solar year, each lunar month moves ten days earlier each year. The start and end of Ramadan is dependent on the sighting of the new moon.

During this month, Muslims fast from pre-dawn until sunset. Muslims fast from food and drink during the daylight hours (which can be anything over twelve hours, depending on where you are in the world) as a means of learning self-control, gratitude and compassion for those less fortunate, and it also allows Muslims to devote themselves to their faith and come closer to God. It is also a time for spiritual reflection, prayer and doing good deeds, such as increased giving to charity. Those unable to fast, such as pregnant or nursing women, the sick, elderly people and children, are exempt from fasting.

At sunset, Muslims break the fast with a few dates and milk or water, and then eat and drink as normal. This is referred to as *iftar* in Arabic. We also eat and drink at *suhoor*, the pre-fast meal, just before dawn.

I choose to continue to run whilst fasting in Ramadan as it's important to me to keep some form of normality and keep doing what I enjoy. During this time, I usually run easier miles at low intensity to decrease the load on my body. I also pay particular attention to what I eat and drink as it's only a small window to provide my body with all the key nutrients that it needs. It's key that I hydrate well and include foods that are rich in complex carbohydrates so that I am still fuelling my body well. In Ramadan there is a tendency to eat more fried food; however, this is something I personally avoid.

The time of day that I run whilst fasting is something to consider too. I choose to run about ninety minutes before sunset, which means that after completing my run I can eat and drink a short while after. This can be hard, as by this point I would have been fasting for over twelve hours and would be at my weakest and most tired, especially when it's summer and it's very warm.

It's also important that I listen to my body, so on days that I'm feeling particularly exhausted I tend to focus on home workouts such as yoga or strength training.

It can affect performance, as I do find I'm more tired. So I focus on easy miles (i.e. no speed work or anything high intensity), slow down my training in terms of distance and intensity, and focus on maintenance. This is a positive, as it gives my body a natural break from training and allows me to recover from periods of high training.

....

PROFESSIONAL OPINION

It is clear to see that Taz has managed to balance her religious beliefs and practices with her love for running and training. While fasting may not be a dietary approach she follows all the time, she has been able to identify the best way to modify her training so that she can continue to run but without additional stress to her body. She has considered the timing of training and how best to recover within Ramadan.

This is a great example of someone who has taken a challenging scenario but made it work for her. She understands that the principle of fasting may not be ideal with regard to the stress it can place on her body, or even the fact that it could hinder her performance, and has learnt to respond to her body day by day.

In this case, fasting is for religious reasons and not for a specific performance or body-composition outcome. This means that Taz can be more objective and listen to her body. However, in those cases where an individual uses IF for a more specific outcome, they may not always be as in sync with their bodies and thus ignore signs that it is under stress.

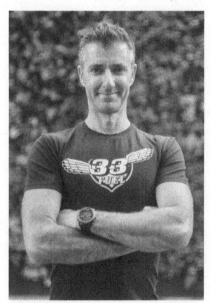

© Filippo Mazzarino

WARREN'S STORY

Warren owns a sports nutrition brand called 33Fuel. He approached me a few years ago to talk on his podcast, initially regarding orthorexia and how it can impact athletes, their health and performance, but then for a second time when I challenged a post his brand did on intermittent fasting. Since then we have continued to chew the fat on a number of sports-nutrition topics.

Having spent the last twelve years as a dedicated amateur endurance athlete focused on ultramarathons and distance triathlons, strength work never much appealed, and given the choice between an hour in the gym or three on the bike or a run, I'd always choose the latter. Strength could come later.

But in the last couple of years, it was obvious my training was becoming unbalanced. While I could run, swim and bike well, everyday strength and flexibility were declining and as my forty-seventh birthday passed I realised 'later' for strength was actually 'now'.

So I slashed my endurance training, swapping much of it for strength work. Even so, three months in, I wasn't seeing results. It's in my nature to look for natural ways to maximise fitness and health – it's one of the major reasons my day job is running the natural sports nutrition company 33Fuel, which my wife Erica and I founded together in 2012 – and so I quizzed all of my expert contacts in the space and researched hard.

Optimising my testosterone levels looked like the best bet, and among the well-tested (and easily implementable) strategies was intermittent fasting, which was as simple as keeping a twelve- to eighteen-hour gap between dinner and breakfast. All I had to do was make sure dinner was around 7 p.m. and the rest looked after itself, while occasional late breakfasts/brunches fitted the plan perfectly too. It also helped with my sleep quality (in itself beneficial to testosterone levels), as I wasn't as hard at work digesting into the small hours as I had been with later dinners.

The gains finally began and in the last twelve months I've added 9 kilograms of lean muscle and feel noticeably stronger, more flexible and generally more resilient. I've also discovered an unexpected enjoyment in lifting heavy(ish) things up and down.

Because I added other strategies as part of my testosterone protocol alongside the intermittent fasting, including – among others – daily maca and creatine supplementation, cold showers and a standing desk to reduce my worktime sitting hours, isolating it as the sole beneficial element isn't possible. However, given the evidence behind it, its ease of implementation and the lack of any downside, I'm not only confident it played a part but I'm also very happy to continue with it.

PROFESSIONAL OPINION

It is very useful having Warren's story as a comparison to Taz's, as someone who has chosen to follow IF. While it is an approach that has resulted in positive outcomes for Warren, he himself alludes to the fact that he can't be sure whether the improvement is due to the IF or one or more of the other changes he made at the same time.

We know that testosterone can decline in males as they get older. Indeed, we discuss this in detail in chapter 8, which is dedicated to the masters athlete. One way to avoid a decline in lean muscle mass as we get older is to include a more structured strength programme. Studies have shown that this has a big impact on reducing muscle mass, which in turn maintains our endurance performance. Interestingly, in the studies that have been conducted on athletes who do IF, two of the key recommendations are that the athlete introduces a resistance programme and also considers increasing protein, still with sufficient carbohydrate, in order to limit loss of lean muscle mass.

Warren has obviously done his research and found a way of eating that works for him, but numerous studies conclude that big gaps in energy distribution during the day, especially if there is an overall low energy availability, contribute to a decline in testosterone. So, Warren needs to be mindful of maintaining a sufficient energy intake. In my professional opinion, the change in lean muscle mass is most likely the cause of improvement in Warren's testosterone levels rather than the IF approach. While he is confident and wants to continue with this approach, my advice would be that he should keep a check on other metabolic parameters such as thyroid function and immune health to ensure no other areas of his health are being affected.

Summary of key points

As a weight-loss strategy, while it is not superior to calorie-controlled approaches, IF may be easier to follow, especially the time-restricted model where food can only be consumed in a specific time window. Similarly, IF may help improve body composition, blood pressure and gut health, although convincing evidence for this latter area is still missing.

There is no evidence to support the idea that IF improves athletic performance. However, some individuals whose focus is weight loss rather than performance may find this approach useful and easier than a restrictive eating pattern. As with all diets, the primary focus should be on providing the athletic body with the nutrients and energy required for both health and performance.

CHAPTER 6

Calorie-Controlled Diets

The concept

A low-calorie, calorie-restricted or calorie-controlled diet is based around a target intake of calories each day. Designed to provide a straightforward way to lose weight, this kind of diet is usually a key method used by weight-loss plans and slimming clubs. As with intermittent fasting, calorie-controlled diets do not restrict the types of food consumed, only the overall calorie value, which will necessarily be an estimate, particularly if you prepare your own food from scratch.

Of the athletes who completed our survey, 16% reported that they had attempted to restrict their nutritional intake while maintaining training in order to lose weight with the aim of improving performance. However, many also reported that their restrictive dietary approaches were not sustainable, generally leading to fatigue and a loss in performance after a period of three to six months.

According to the Health Survey for England 2019, 28% of adults were defined as obese and a further 36% overweight, but how do these figures relate to an active or athletic population?[25] The criterion used to determine this data was BMI, body mass index, which is the ratio between your height and weight. BMI has come under a lot of scrutiny in recent years as it doesn't consider body composition. Indeed, this is a fact that many athletes and sports also do not take into account – often, as we stated above, focusing on achieving a specific weight, rather than appreciating the importance of lean muscle mass on performance. Body composition is an important parameter in both the athlete and non-athlete population because fat-free mass – that is, lean muscle mass – is a lot more metabolically active than fat mass, but while it may take up less space than body fat, it does weigh more. If you cast your mind back to chapter 1 where we discussed how large deficits in energy taken in compared with energy expended may lead to a reduced body mass in people who are overweight and/or obese, often these losses are short-lived and not maintained unless body composition is improved.

There are many advantages to health of maintaining body-fat percentage within normal parameters. In females this will be a range of 21–30%, and in males 14–24%, with higher-level athletes often sitting a little lower. Female athletes tend to be around 14–21%, while male athletes can be 6–14%, depending on the sport. However, it is important to highlight here that in order for females to be fertile – that is, they have regular menstruation – body-fat percentage usually needs to be a minimum of 17% in teenagers and 21% in adults. Thus, many female athletes in particular may need to periodise their body composition around competition for optimal health and performance, rather than aiming for an unsustainably and unhealthily lean body composition throughout the year, to avoid longer-term damage to reproductive and bone health.

Pros and cons

Calorie-controlled diets sound easy, but the reality can be far from it. Suggested calorie intakes must be low enough to induce a negative energy balance in order to lose weight, but not by too much so as to trigger compensatory mechanisms such as lowering BMR (basal metabolic rate). As we discussed in chapter 1, however, accurately calculating how much energy an individual expends each day is difficult, and depends on many factors. Restrictive diets are often unpleasant to undertake, leading to obsessing about food, low mood and difficulty concentrating.

It's worth considering whether restricting calories is necessary, or whether changes in diet composition or habits might be more effective. Additionally, while some recreational athletes will have a genuine need to lose weight for health and improving performance, others (possibly erroneously) believe weight loss will give them a performance edge.

BEING SELF-AWARE

Many of us will turn to exercise as a method of trying to lose weight, improve health metrics or manage our mental health, and there is a lot of evidence that demonstrates how movement can benefit our mental well-being, but there is a big difference between movement, exercise and training. There are also those of us, albeit in the minority, who turn to exercise as a way of attaining worth or coping with a lack of confidence and self-esteem. This is not a conscious stream of thought or process, but something that may become evident once you start training. While I'm not saying it will affect everyone, having self-awareness around your relationship with exercise is important to stop it becoming a 'coping mechanism' and a dysfunctional behaviour.

Where does this all come from? Why the constant need and search for 'perfect'?

It does feel as though we are a society that defines individuals by external validation. We are only deemed successful if we have 'achieved'. There is constant pressure to live by ideals, from what we look like to what we eat, even to how the interior of our home looks.

In athletes, the highly competitive environment creates the need to constantly push and prove their place, often to the detriment of their long-term health. It feels like we live in a constant state of judgement. For those of us who are vulnerable and who struggle with our sense of self, this creates more anxiety. We crack the whip harder, but no matter what we do, we are never good enough. While love and happiness are positive emotions to experience, many of us run a mile (quite literally) when it comes to experiencing difficult emotions such as loss, rejection, pain, criticism and trauma. Indeed, human beings are hard-wired to avoid threat.

It's understandable because, as many of us who suffer with anxiety know, it can be debilitating. It's those severe physical feelings that you can sense deep within you, making you want to just unzip and escape from your body. However, the problem is that no matter what 'coping mechanisms' you put in place to 'control, contain and numb' these difficult emotions, such as restrictive eating, over-exercising, alcohol, sex or drugs, they are always temporary.

How we navigate these difficult emotions will often depend on how they were handled in our childhood. Were negative experiences brushed under the carpet, or did we learn that disappointment and failure is part of the human experience? Did we come from an environment that taught us about conditional acceptance – that we are only worthy of care, attention and approval if we achieve – rather than unconditional? In this way, we learn to attain worth through different means, such as sporting success, academic achievement or our image. In comparison, unconditional acceptance is where we learn to show up for ourselves and provide reassurance, compassion and care, even if the outcome/response didn't work out the way we had wanted or hoped.

Case studies and discussion

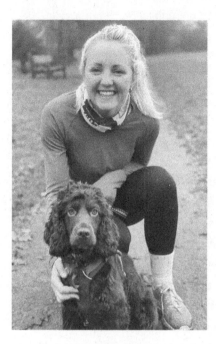

HANNAH'S STORY

Hannah and I met over social media. She is one half of Twice the Health, a running blog/platform. She actually contacted me as they wanted me to do a talk for them on nutrition, running and RED-S. On the back of this, Hannah contacted me personally for some support. Since then, we have become firm friends and work together in a number of capacities, always trying to raise awareness on RED-S and how to achieve more of a balance towards training and health.

I was not the usual suspect, or at least I didn't think I was. I'd fortunately never suffered with any kind of difficult relationship with food: I ate all day every day and believed I was putting enough in my body. I didn't track, but I always made an effort to eat relatively well to allow myself to continue to train for the endurance sports I loved. Or at least I thought so.

Whilst training for my first single-stage ultra, I missed a period. I'd always been very regular, and never had any fluctuation with time of the month. I put it down to stress until it happened again, at which point I reached out to Renee. We went through my food diary and discovered that since switching to a more vegetarian-based diet, when the food company I worked for launched said package, I had been unknowingly getting a lot of my carbs from vegetable sources, as opposed to my usual rice/pasta/bread, simply due to how the meals were structured. Naively, I hadn't thought anything of it, but once pointed out it made sense. Renee advised me to add extra rice to the meals delivered and be more aware of getting bread-based snacks in where possible. Within three months my periods were back to normal.

I was one of the lucky ones, educated enough to reach out and fortunate enough to suffer no psychological effects. I'm so grateful to Renee for being there.

....

PROFESSIONAL OPINION

RED-S is not always a result of a conscious decision to restrict your energy intake. There are numerous cases where it occurs accidentally. Lifestyle and training levels are so active that the individual doesn't always appreciate just how much fuel their body requires to operate optimally. In Hannah's case, her workload and intensity were high, especially as she was training for a specific event; and while her energy intake was good, her overall carbohydrate availability was low in comparison. As Hannah says, she has never had any difficulties with her relationship with food and exercise, so rectifying this situation was easy. I provided her with the information she required, she put it into practice and within a very short time her periods returned.

It can be very difficult to fully appreciate the amount of fuel your body requires, especially as we live in an era where we are always being told to 'move more and eat less'. While we know a large percentage of the UK population is overweight and/or obese, it is important to be able to appreciate that not all public-health messaging is relevant to you. If you are an athlete or someone who is physically very active, maintaining energy intake may prove to be challenging. As we have seen, RED-S can occur in anyone who participates in sport – any level, any stage, any age and any gender. Being mindful of the symptoms and acting on them as soon as possible can help to ensure no long-lasting damage is done to health and performance.

....

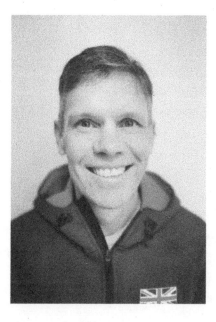

JAMES'S STORY

James and I first met at the 24-Hour (running) World Championships in Belfast. He was representing GB and I had been asked to come along to crew and also provide general support to the whole team. Post-Belfast, James and I started working together specifically on his performance nutrition, and in recent years he has gone on to become a huge support and mentor to me and my work.

Nutrition – huh! It was an afterthought for me. I actually ran chiefly to offset a diet that was pizza, chips, crisps and chocolate. Then in 2011 I decided to get serious about running, to see what I could achieve. Little did I know by 2016 I would be representing Scotland and Great Britain at ultra distance and winning races on multiple continents. In 2011 I was almost four stone heavier than I would get to by the time I was running for my country.

If you asked me to pinpoint the key things that made the difference for me, it would be quality of training, looking after my body with stretching and mobility and, most crucially, my nutrition.

Prior to 2014 – and it is horrific to write this – I had never eaten a salad in my life. All that effort for so few calories. I thought calories was the one and only currency that mattered when it came to fuel-in. Then I got to reading about the part quality fuel played in both performance and recovery. Renee's *Training Food* was a key catalyst in my change to better eating. It can seem almost incomprehensible to some that I could be so ignorant of the importance of a quality diet, but growing up I was so fussy my folks would just be happy I was eating something, anything. At one stage I was nearly referred for being too skinny as a young kid, so consumption became the key. Quantity over quality. That habit is something I still have to be mindful of today.

There are clearly some obvious benefits to having broadened my palate. My body-fat percentage plummeted, yet my weight has been less yo-yo. I find my recovery is exceptional as I know what mix of protein, carbs and nutrients to have before, during and after big efforts. And a big effort to me in training can be forty- to fifty-mile runs. In 2017 I went full vegetarian. This forced me to be more adventurous in my eating. I have discovered foods that would have sounded like magic spells to pre-2011 James!

Equally as important, my performances improved markedly. Since 2015 I have won ultras and marathons every year, often multiple races. I represented Scotland in 2016 and 2019. I represented Great Britain in 2017, 2018 and 2019, and missed out on running for GB in 2020 and 2021 due to Covid.

Aligning my eating to my training to my ambitions was a critical step in my athlete life. Without it, I'd be decent but never realise my potential. With it, I have been able to find levels of achievement I never dreamed possible. I feel, look and am healthier as a result. If that isn't motivation enough, then I don't know what is.

I have never been a slave to my nutrition. I control it and, for those reading, balance is critical. I still enjoy pizza, just at the right times now! It's not about being obsessive; it is about being aware and making better choices. And I try to do this every day now.

....

PROFESSIONAL OPINION

James's story is a breath of fresh air and demonstrates how it wasn't over-restriction and creating huge deficits that improved his body composition and performance, but educating himself about how to fuel his training appropriately.

All too often, individuals focus on the number on the scales as being the focused outcome and this then creates poor habits: dietary over-restriction while also trying to train at high volumes, with a mantra of 'move more, eat less' ringing in their ears but usually ending in defeat and then weight piling back on, or injury and illness.

Making appropriate choices around your training, resulting in a small deficit, is the most sustainable way of not only losing weight, but also achieving health and performance.

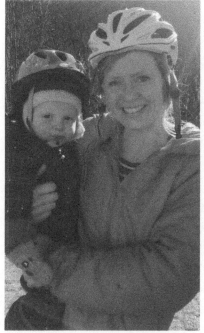

© Stuart Duggan

MINA'S STORY

Mina was a client who self-referred to my clinic that I jointly run with a consultant endocrinologist. She has a long-standing history of primary amenorrhoea due to the extremes she placed her body under for her sport. While highly successful for the most part of her career, in recent years she had noticed that, no matter what she did, her body no longer responded. In addition, she was keen to start to consider having a family and so wanted support and advice with her menstrual health.

Rock climbing has always been a huge part of my life. From competitions to outdoor adventures, it has been a constant source of happiness, fun, challenge and connection. I started when I was just a little girl of eight and was hooked immediately; as such, being now a thirty-four-year-old woman, I almost don't remember life without it.

Of course, during this time there have been setbacks and moments of difficulty. I stepped back from climbing for some short phases during the

95

last twenty-six years due to various injuries (broken bones, sprains and a nasty head injury), but the greatest personal challenge for me came in the form of Relative Energy Deficiency in Sport.

Climbing is, without a doubt, a weight-sensitive sport. This means that how heavy an athlete is relative to their strength affects their ability to move up a rock face. The problem is that climbing culture focuses far too much on the weight, and not enough on the strength. This desire for lightness combined with a 'more is more' approach to training and exercise led me to a diagnosis of hypothalamic amenorrhoea (loss of menstrual cycle). My body was in a state of low energy availability from over-exercising (climbing, running, swimming, etc.) and not fuelling enough to meet the demands of my activity levels. Part of the problem was how much I loved doing all these things. The other, darker side was a gradual fixation on being lighter and lighter. It's worth mentioning that I was never 'underweight', and this gave me a false sense of security that my health could not possibly be compromised. Oh, how wrong I was. With low energy, creeping fatigue, loss of menstruation (and temporarily my fertility), vulnerable bones and an inability to keep warm, I was far from the picture of health.

The diagnosis from Renee and Nicky was a huge shock and it took me some time to process what it meant moving forward. I continued to climb and run initially while increasing my food intake, in particular carbohydrates. Over the first few months, I gained weight fast – it was like my body was desperate to hold onto everything. This was really difficult for me psychologically; my performance plummeted, I struggled with body image and I lost confidence. At this point, the Intuitive Eating Framework helped me hugely to trust my body and give it time. But still there was no sign of my period.

The final commitment was full rest, and, for me, this was the hardest part but also the most fruitful. I stopped everything activity-wise apart from easy walks and carried on eating what felt like everything. After a couple more months, my period returned. A few months later, I returned gradually to climbing with a focus on fuelling well, resting enough and honouring my body. I saw strength gains that in the past had eluded me, and I finally saw that it might be possible to be a better athlete at a heavier weight. My return to form was interrupted again, but this time in a positive way – I fell pregnant. My initial diagnosis had scared me so much as I had always wanted children, so this was a huge motivator for my recovery.

Now I am eight weeks post-partum and navigating my return to climbing. I hope that the next twenty-five years are full of fun, challenge and connection, but with more patience, respect and knowledge of my body.

PROFESSIONAL OPINION

Mina's story is not unique, sadly. Every day in clinic, I hear a similar version of the above events. Mina was brave and proactive in getting help, maybe because she knew she wanted to have a family one day. She took on board the advice and, while it was not easy, she used the same determined athlete mindset to sit with the discomfort, which resulted in a very happy ending.

However, many athletes struggle with modifying their diet and training. They find it difficult to challenge their limiting beliefs around weight and performance, which means they stay stuck in a cycle of destruction, poor performance and deteriorating health.

Acknowledging you need help is the first step, followed by sourcing the appropriate support.

Summary of key points

We can see that restrictive intakes do not work for athletes. In most cases, they lead to poor performance and extreme fatigue, which is usually enough for the athlete to abort this practice.

In some cases, athletes develop very strong beliefs that can lead to a phenomenon known as RED-S, which can have detrimental impact on both health and performance. These individuals need to work with specialist practitioners to help reverse and restore their bodies.

Recovery from RED-S

We have seen from the literature, and also from Mina's account, that RED-S doesn't always result in weight loss. As stated earlier, this is because of the body's compensatory mechanisms, which, among other effects, slow metabolic rate to conserve energy.

This can make it difficult not only to diagnose but also to identify. An athlete becomes more and more frustrated when their body mass does not change, even though in their mind they are training harder and restricting their intake. While the body will sustain this for a period, chronic under-fuelling and low energy availability results in stagnation and then deterioration in performance and health.

Women are more sensitive to low energy availability due to the higher demands of their reproductive systems. When the hypothalamus detects that there is not sufficient energy to sustain a potential pregnancy, it shuts down the hormones associated with menstruation. This is usually one of the first signs in a female that they are under-fuelling. However, an important caveat is that this is not the only sign and, in some women, there is a sub-clinical picture where a bleed still occurs but it is known as an anovulatory period: the individual is not ovulating but the slight change in hormones means they still shed their uterine lining to give a 'bleed'.

While male athletes are impacted by low energy availability, it may take slightly longer for signs to become apparent, especially those associated with production of sex hormones. In fact, by the time a male athlete notices that changes are occurring, their testosterone levels will be very low, less than 10 micromoles per litre. Healthy males should expect levels in the mid-twenties, while most endurance athletes will sit somewhere in the high teens. Low levels of testosterone usually manifest in a loss of morning erectile function on at least five days per week.

As previously mentioned, RED-S can be difficult to recognise, and it involves clinical and psychological assessment of the individual's relationship with food, training and body image, along with blood tests that can rule out any other medical condition. One thing to note when doing blood tests, especially in female athletes, is that these will be disguised if they are on certain types of contraception. Therefore, careful questioning and working with highly trained practitioners is critical.

The tests that we specifically look at include reproductive hormones, thyroid hormones, vitamin D, iron, white cell count and the stress hormone cortisol. In general, all of these will be down-regulated, so not necessarily out of range but on the very low end of the normal range, with the exception being cortisol, which tends to be high.

Thus, one of the key aspects of recovery from RED-S is restoration of biochemical and hormonal health. This can be achieved through modification to training and addressing not only low energy availability, but also the composition and timing of nutrition.

Weight loss is achievable if it needs to be and is done in a sustainable manner. That said, the number on the scales should not be the focus. Using different outcomes such as health metrics and girth measurements can be a more helpful and healthy way to improve body composition and performance.

PART 2

Fuelling for Specific Populations

In this second part of the book, my aim is to provide
information on areas within sports science that may
often be neglected but are highly significant.

CHAPTER 7

The Female
Athlete

Introduction

Participation in sport increased in both men and women during 2019–2020, pre-pandemic. During this time frame, the Active Lives adult survey reported that 61% of women were active, that is doing 150+ minutes of moderate physical activity or 75 minutes of vigorous physical activity per week; 13% were moderately active (30–149 minutes a week); and 26% were inactive.[26] According to recent data, there has been a slow and steady increase in the number of women who participate in any kind of sport or physical activity in the UK. In England in 2021, approximately 17.5 million women (75%) participated at least twice a month at any intensity or duration, a slight decrease from 17.78 million women in 2020.[27]

In competitive sports, women's participation is gradually increasing, with women making up nearly half of London Marathon applicants (48% in 2020). London Marathon event director Hugh Brasher observed that, 'At the first London Marathon back in 1981, fewer than 300 of the 6,300 finishers were women. More than 179,000 women from the UK have applied to run in 2020.'[28]

While sports based around physical size, strength and power are always likely to be dominated by men, particularly at the highest level, recent years have seen female athletes starting to work their way through the field in ultra-distance events. High overall placings and even overall wins by women are becoming commonplace, with recent successes by Jasmin Paris, Courtney Dauwalter and Beth Pascall; and in 2021 an incredible fifteen of the top thirty finishers at the Western States 100 ultramarathon were women. It's likely this is due to the numerous additional factors involved in such events, including, from a physical perspective, women being better able to utilise body fat for fuel, and the advantage of larger, more powerful muscles being less important over longer distances, along with the other aspects of ultra-distance races such as self-care and meticulous pre-race preparation.

Sport and the menstrual cycle

Many of us are familiar with the monthly fluctuations in hormones that can affect the way we feel and experience the world from one day to the next. But hormonal variations can also have a significant effect on our sport, from changes in mood and motivation to aspects of physical (dis) comfort and how we choose to fuel our bodies.

The menstrual cycle affects everyone differently, but for the majority of people who menstruate, there will be some impact of hormonal changes on training and competition. Understanding this can not only help you manage your training better, but it can also ensure that you make the right choices for fuel on race day. Most importantly, it also stops you from beating yourself up when the numbers don't stack up, and when the only food group that exists in your diet is chocolate.

While a regular menstrual cycle can be anything from twenty-two to forty days, the average cycle is twenty-eight days and there can be monthly variations of a few days. What is essential to understand is that there will be a 'normal' for you, and if your cycle changes significantly by becoming much shorter or longer, this may be your body trying to tell you something.

The menstrual cycle and its resulting changes and uncertainties are a large part of the reason why women are traditionally under-represented in scientific research. Indeed, a lot of the scientific literature in female athletes is done in those who are on the combined oral contraceptive pill, as this helps to standardise hormonal environments. What we do know is that, in the same way as no two women have the same menstrual cycle, no two women are going to have the same symptoms. Hormones are constantly changing and, while you may notice that training and life in general feels a bit harder at certain times of the month, this can also fluctuate over a year. Maybe this is why it is so difficult to get a full understanding of how hormones influence us on a daily, weekly and monthly basis. For this reason, we have to look at trends but also keep an open mind; we cannot ignore the impact of lifestyle and daily stress that will also play a role in how we feel.

The menstrual cycle

In general, it is important to remember that you are most likely to be unaffected by your cycle in the early phase (see overleaf for a summary of the phases), although that said, being aware and mindful of your nutritional intake around the mid-follicular phase seems to be critical for ovulation to occur. This is heightened in women who have a history of chronically low energy availability, as even once this has been restored, their menstrual cycle is still sensitive to change in energy and carbohydrate availability. Similarly, post-ovulation, during the second half of your cycle, you may notice more changes in core temperature, blood-sugar fluctuations and cravings, as well as changes to mood. The severity of your symptoms does seem to be related to how high your progesterone levels rise and then have to fall to return to baseline figures, which again is very individual and most likely genetic.

Phase 1

Days 1–7, with day 1 being the first day of your menstrual period. This is known as the follicular phase.

- Oestrogen and progesterone are at low levels.

Phase 2

Days 8–14, still within follicular phase but ovulation occurs around day 10–12.

- Oestrogen rising, peaking just before ovulation.

- Blood sugars are more stable and, due to the higher levels of oestrogen, the body becomes more efficient at using fat for fuel, but this doesn't mean you should reduce your intake of carbohydrate.

- You may even find your training feels a little easier.

Phase 3

Days 15–21, just post-ovulation, now within the luteal phase.

- Both oestrogen and progesterone begin to rise.

- The effect of your progesterone impacts your BMR, which then starts to rise, so you may recognise an increase in appetite and cravings.

- You may notice an elevated heart rate during training and at rest, as well as an increase in temperature and sweat. Be mindful of this during this phase, and train off heart rate as opposed to pace.

Phase 4

Days 22–28, the luteal phase, premenstrual.

- Oestrogen and progesterone start to fall to their lowest point, ready for menses.

- Increased appetite and cravings are likely. Sleep can also become fractious, which can affect recovery, concentration, alertness and overall performance.

- Stress and anxiety can impact PMS.

- This is the point in the cycle where it's more important than ever to listen to what your body can do and focus on training for well-being rather than for performance.

- When oestrogen is low and rising, we are more efficient at using fat as a fuel source, especially during moderate-intensity training. While carbohydrates are still necessary for exercise, we will also use a higher percentage of fat for fuel, meaning we are likely to feel so much stronger in training and racing. Our mood is also more likely to be more stable and rational.

- However, as progesterone rises, our blood sugars fluctuate a lot more, and we rely on carbohydrate for fuel during our training. In general, our body is working harder at this stage, which is why the same training, whether it's an easy run or an interval turbo session, is going to feel so much harder.

- From a nutrient-specific point of view, women who have heavier periods, and thus higher menstrual losses, may need to keep an eye on their iron intake, especially if they are physically active.

- If you are competing during your luteal phase, you will need to keep carbohydrate stores topped up to maintain optimal performance. During this stage, our bodies are also very inefficient at using stored carbohydrate as a fuel source, so your extrinsic carbohydrate source is going to be important, especially during endurance events. We would typically recommend 30–60 grams of carbohydrates per hour for events up to three hours, and 60–90 grams of carbohydrate per hour in events over three hours, where you will need to be taking on closer to the upper end to maintain the pace.

- So, while you can use the above phases as general guidelines, the key is to monitor your own cycles and start to work out what your personal fluctuations and trends are.

The effect of the menstrual cycle on physical performance is currently a popular topic in sport science literature. A 2021 narrative review explored the findings of a number of studies investigating the effects of menstrual cycle phase on both athletes' perceived and objectively measured performance, concluding:

Studies examining perceived performance consistently report that female athletes identify their performance to be relatively worse during the early follicular and late luteal phases. Studies examining objective performance (using anaerobic, aerobic or strength-related tests) do not report clear, consistent effects of the impact of menstrual cycle phase on physical performance.[29]

So, while it is valuable to know that our objective performance isn't necessarily going to be negatively impacted by our menstrual cycle, it's also important to fully acknowledge the role of perceived performance, including aspects such as pain, discomfort and the practicalities of managing bleeding during menstruation, as well as the fluctuations in mood and motivation that may occur throughout the cycle.

Why have my periods stopped?

Sometimes, the frequency, flow or occurrence of periods can change, and, in athletes and active people, this can be related to energy availability. If change is consistent, then it is always advised to seek medical help. Some common medical causes include:

- **Polycystic ovary syndrome (PCOS)**
  This would need to be confirmed by blood tests and/or ultrasound, looking at both the lining of the uterus and the potential development of cysts. Also, there should be other non-menstrual clinical symptoms such as acne. Something to be mindful of is that many women are told they have PCOS when it is clear they have hypothalamic amenorrhoea because of low energy availability or RED-S. This usually occurs when the woman in question is of normal weight, and it is assumed that she must be fuelling appropriately. However, it is often the case that history and relationship with food and/or training are rarely asked about.

- **Pregnancy**

- **Breastfeeding**
  As a result of breastfeeding, the body will produce high levels of prolactin, which temporarily stop menstruation, but this is generally only when breastfeeding is exclusive. As breastfeeding reduces, periods are likely to return, but each time frame will be individual.

- **Hormonal contraception**
  The combined oral contraceptive pill down-regulates the hypothalamus and so stops ovulation from occurring. While many women believe they are having a period when they are on the pill, they are not. This is a withdrawal bleed and may mask symptoms of low energy availability such as hypothalamic amenorrhoea.

What is hypothalamic amenorrhoea?

While the above are medical reasons why your period may stop or become erratic, if these causes have been excluded then we use the term hypothalamic amenorrhoea. If periods have not started before the age of sixteen years, this is known as primary amenorrhoea. For women who have had an established menstrual cycle prior to them stopping, we call this secondary amenorrhoea, but only when this exceeds six months. That said, the loss of three consecutive periods should ring alarm bells and medical advice should be sought as soon as possible.

One point to raise here is that there is no such thing as post-contraception amenorrhoea. While it may take up to six or eight weeks maximum for hormones to regulate after ceasing hormonal contraception, beyond this a lack of menstruation needs to be investigated.

The most common cause of amenorrhoea is when there is not sufficient energy availability to do the work required by the body. 'Work' covers all physical activity, including training as well as day-to-day activities such as walking to the bus stop or brushing your teeth. On top of this, it also includes work that the body does in terms of biological processes such as hormonal regulation, digestion, immune and bone health.

The common factors that may contribute to this are:

- overtraining
- high-intensity training in a fasted state
- under-fuelling, either intentionally or unintentionally
- the athlete mentality leading to restrictive eating and exercise dependency
- rapid weight loss, again either intentionally or unintentionally
- food trends, particularly those that involve fasting or removing carbohydrates.

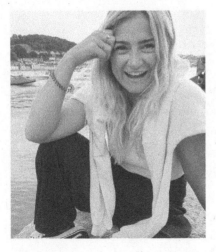

CHLO'S STORY

Chlo came to my clinic for support. She had not had a period for a while and was also aware that her relationship with food and exercise was not healthy. Over the course of several months, with nutrition, exercise modification and behavioural interventions, she eventually overcame her hypothalamic amenorrhoea.

I'm still to this day not sure how long I actually had HA for, as I was on the pill for around seven or eight years before I came off it and my period didn't return. I know for certain that my disordered relationship with food and exercise had started a few years before I came off the pill.

I started running as a way to get fit at fifteen after being called a slob by an ex-boyfriend, and it became my therapy. It was that thirty minutes of 'me' time when I could sometimes cry or, most of the time, just switch off. Soon after, I started fitness classes, and that's where my toe tapped into the fitness industry. I was introduced to fasted cardio, calories, different types of exercise, people doing back-to-back gym classes, low-carb, low-fat, juice cleanses. Wow! 'I could fit in here,' I remember thinking.

I remember doing ab workout DVDs in my bedroom after having done two classes in the gym, just to do a little extra. I started eating lots of protein, lots of dry chicken and veggies (that's what the others did, right?); chocolate became a no and carbs a never. I started telling people that I just didn't like bread or rice so I could avoid eating them. The body checking in the mirror became more of a thing and the happiness deepened.

I got so caught up in trying to be perfect, to be good enough and slim enough, that I wanted to try everything. I started laxatives, I tried clen (can't remember the full name), I tried cardio in the morning and HIIT in the evening. I was eating under 1,000 calories a day and if I went to bed hungry, then that was a pat on the back.

Yet everyone just thought I was the healthy one, the fit one – and I did, too. I loved it.

Soon after, I was introduced to calorie counting after training to be a PT and doing a nutrition for aesthetics course. Wow, I could eat so much more! But my obsession to be perfect and good enough soon became something I could quantify: 'Hit that number, never any more, but if you want to go lower then you'll only lose more weight.'

Then came the rise of Instagram: SO.MUCH.FITNESS. I tried everything, all the classes. I used to come to London just to go to fitness classes. I was sucked right in and looked at everyone in the classes and on Instagram to see how I could be just like them!

I was consumed by not feeling good enough and being so unhappy that I was trying to find the answer within my body.

I eventually decided to end things with an on-off boyfriend of seven to eight years at twenty-two and that was the start of my journey of self-discovery. I booked Australia and Thailand and got offered a dream job as a content producer. It was so exciting and so liberating, I came off the pill and my period didn't return.

I had come across Renee's work before from Natacha Océane, and I had seen that Sarah's Day lost her period too, so I was aware. I won't lie,

I was proud that I also fitted into that category of my two favourite YouTubers (my heart breaks for my old self). I started looking into it more and realised I needed to eat more and train less (potentially), but I couldn't. It was my safe place, my comfort zone – and now I thought if I stopped, people wouldn't fancy me or like me. I had a reputation of 'the gym one' to keep up!

I dived into education and read more and more and more. I slowly started making very small, controlled changes – I ate a little more food and did a little less HIIT.

I went to the doctor, who told me I was absolutely fine, it was common and to come back in three months. This went on for around nine months before I demanded to be referred to a gynaecologist. They weighed me and congratulated me on my weight as it's not often they get people not overweight in there. I tried to speak to all of them about exercise and my food problems and they said, 'Okay, exercise less and maybe eat a little more to fuel your exercise, but you're a great weight so don't worry … oh, and you might have PCOS.' Really?

Five minutes later she came back in the room and said, 'I've just spoken to [someone above her] and he has confirmed you don't have PCOS, so we aren't really sure as your hormones all seem fine and scan is good. So, we'd recommend you go on the pill, so I'll sort that for you now.'

'Oh. I'm fine? The pill? No thanks, I know this is just a plaster and not sorting it.'

'Well, this is what we'd recommend.'

They dismissed me, saying they wouldn't work with me further unless I wanted kids and I should go on the pill to have my period back.

I left in floods of tears. 'WHAT IS WRONG WITH ME?' I remember shouting at myself in the car mirror. 'Is this really my world now? IBS, poor skin, low mood, reliant on caffeine, constantly bloated and waking up in the night? No sex drive … I really do ruin everything I touch, don't I?'

My family still thought I was the healthy one. I went back for some more blood work and my doctor mentioned something about my kidneys not working as well. This was when Mum was like, 'Oh my God, okay, we need to take this seriously now,' and I told her about Renee. I booked my appointment in the December and because of the amazing work she does, had my appointment in the March. One week before the first lockdown.

Renee changed my life. She confirmed all my issues, all my problems I knew I had and confirmed my hormones weren't in fact okay. She listened, spoke about where it stemmed from and set me a plan.

Fortunately, my poor attempt at getting better had benefitted me as my hormones weren't completely non-existent, but I made some huge changes and put all my trust in Renee. I started eating more and following her plan. It was hard, but I think living alone in lockdown helped me – for someone who always looked for external validation, I only had me to deal with. I worked through feeling good enough as I am, completely changing my lifestyle and mindset.

I had a follow-up session with Renee after a little freak-out about six weeks in but Renee just reassured me and talked things through with me and continued to offer support until I was confident that my menstruation had returned consistently, and that is something I'm forever grateful for. Renee always says, 'I'm just doing my job,' but she genuinely helped me (and so many others) change their lives, so it's so much more than just a job in my eyes.

My journey has inspired me to share it across Instagram because when I first realised I had a problem, I wasn't an athlete like Natacha and a lot of people who Renee worked with, and I wasn't ill enough to be classed as having an eating disorder. I was just a regular fitness girl, trying to find perfection. It breaks my heart that there are others out there too doing this to themselves.

My relationship with food is what I would call neutral. Realising there are no 'good' or 'bad' foods was life-changing; realising I could eat chocolate and not wake up 60 stone heavier was a gift from God; and realising that I don't need to exercise every day to be a good person has meant I've finally been able to achieve things I could never even dream of (partly because my head was always focused on the next piece of chicken I'd allow myself to eat).

I genuinely feel free now. Freedom has always been a big thing for me and with the help of Renee I was able to see that freedom was an inside job, with the right guidance and information I was able to create myself freedom.

I now say I eat mindfully: most of what will do my body good nutritionally with a bit of what my soul wants. I train mindfully too.

....

PROFESSIONAL OPINION

Sadly, Chlo's story is all too familiar these days. What starts out as 'a way of improving myself' soon turns into dysfunctional and obsessive behaviours with health consequences. Thankfully, Chlo knew it was not right for a woman to not have a period if they are not pregnant or breastfeeding. She also knew that going back on the pill was not the answer. She put all the hard work in – looked at her nutrition, modified her training and trusted the process. It sounds simple but, as she has articulated, she has had to challenge and change her mindset. Modern society sets many of us to believe we are not worthy; that we are defined by our image or successes. Learning to build a compassionate and accepting relationship with yourself is a big part of the journey, but it takes time, patience and resilience.

....

From my experience of working with athletes of all levels – recreational through to Olympic and Paralympic standard, young to old, male and female – it is a bit like walking on a tightrope. Stay balanced, and you will make it to the other side; but be aware, it doesn't take much to push this off-kilter.

We live in a society that is always demanding, that requires us to prove our worth through our achievements. For athletes, this will be through sporting success. While healthy competition doesn't hurt anyone, when it becomes something that creates anxiety and defines your worth, it can be something destructive and dysfunctional. This pursuit of 'constant happiness/success/completeness' often results in extreme behaviours, which can result in short- and long-term health problems.

While the culture within sport may suggest that it is normal for active women to lose their periods, we have substantial scientific evidence that demonstrates while it may be a popular occurrence, it has significant consequences to long- and short-term health, as well as a deterioration in performance.

Recovery from hypothalamic amenorrhoea

Recovery from hypothalamic amenorrhoea is complex and involves a number of key considerations:

- Exercise load and intensity
- Body weight and specifically composition
- Overall energy intake, but specifically carbohydrate availability
- Stress, physical and emotional

All these components contribute towards HA. Some women may be affected by all of them, and others perhaps just one or two.

Evaluation of blood tests, taking a comprehensive history of training, nutritional intake and weight/body composition are all critical when deciding on the best intervention and strategies to support women to help restore menstruation. So, it is not as simple as saying you must eat a certain number of calories, or reach a certain weight, before hormonal regulation will return, as we saw from the section on RED-S in chapter 1.

Recovery takes time and, once again, every woman will be different. A lot will depend on the length of time someone has been maintaining the behaviours that have resulted in an absence of their period. Equally, it also depends on where they are at presently with regard to their ability and commitment to change. I've worked with women where it has taken as little as six weeks, to as long as two and a half years. The key is trusting the process.

In some women, where it is clear that bone density has been impacted due to a prolonged period of time with low oestrogen levels, and that it may take time to change certain beliefs and behaviours, hormone replacement therapy should be considered. The Endocrine Society guidelines suggest this as a short-term treatment, no longer than six months, in order to protect bones from any further deterioration while encouraging the individual to work towards achieving her own periods.

For women with a normal (for them), healthy and regular menstrual cycle, logging perceived levels of motivation and performance alongside objective training measures will help to track individual requirements over time.

Fuelling exercise through pregnancy and breastfeeding

In general, we know that being physically active has huge benefits in reducing risk of certain illnesses as well as improving a wide range of physical and mental health metrics. This is no different during pregnancy and breastfeeding. While research is limited, the studies that are available demonstrate not only the benefits but also the importance of trying to stay physically active during pregnancy. Similarly, a 2020 study reported that exercising when breastfeeding increases a compound within breast milk that reduces a baby's lifelong risks of serious health issues such as diabetes, obesity and heart disease.[30]

The present recommendations for exercise during pregnancy include encouraging those who have not been previously active to move moderately for about thirty minutes a day; while those who have always been active should continue to be so, although they may need to be mindful of high-intensity exercise.

After pregnancy, those who are able to do so should work with a pelvic-floor specialist physiotherapist who can ensure that their body is ready to return to training but also provide guidance on how much and how quickly they can progress.

Nutritional guidelines in pregnancy tend to follow those encouraged for the rest of the population: basing meals around complex carbohydrates, including good sources of lean protein, a daily mix and diversity of fruit and vegetables, essential fatty acids, some dairy, and keeping highly processed and sugary foods to a minimum. In addition, eating regularly with good distribution of energy through the day can reduce common pregnancy symptoms such as nausea and constipation. There is a slight increase in energy requirements of around 300 calories a day throughout pregnancy, but the old wives' tale of 'eating for two' no longer stands. For those women who come from an athletic background, as would be the case when not pregnant, energy requirements will be higher when compared to their sedentary peers. The same principles regarding carbohydrate availability and post-training recovery options are important to maintain.

Contrary to what you may have read, an active lifestyle does not affect the quality or amount of breast milk you produce. However, consuming enough energy from nutrient-dense foods along with sufficient fluid will help meet the demands of both breastfeeding and athletic training.

Even without exercise, mothers who breastfeed need extra calories. Calorie needs depend on a variety of factors, including your baby's age and how much you breastfeed. The amount of energy needed for milk production can range from an additional 400 to 500 calories each day when compared to calorie needs prior to pregnancy. In addition, you will also need to consider the amount of energy required based on the duration and intensity of your session.

Fluid needs increase during breastfeeding, too. Without exercise, breastfeeding mothers need about two to three litres of fluid per day from food, beverages and drinking water. Those who add training into the mix will also need to consider their fluid losses associated with exercise.

If you continue to breastfeed after your baby is six months old, you may need to pay attention to your intake of calcium, iron and vitamin D in particular, as your baby will have obtained these from you and your breast milk.

Fuelling training and competition through the menopause

Perimenopause or menopause transition begins several years prior to menopause. It usually starts in a woman's forties but can start earlier in some cases, and can last anything from a few months to ten years. Perimenopause stops at menopause, where the ovaries no longer produce any eggs and oestrogen levels are low.

As there is a great deal of hormonal fluctuation during this time, perimenopause is difficult to detect through blood tests. Common symptoms of perimenopause will vary from woman to woman, but are indicative of what is going on hormonally.

Common signs include:

- lower sex drive
- hot flushes
- worsening premenstrual symptoms
- fatigue
- irregular periods
- vaginal dryness and discomfort during sex
- urinary urgency
- urinary leakage when coughing or sneezing
- mood swings
- increased anxiety and low mood
- trouble sleeping.

It is possible to get all the above or just one or two; there doesn't seem to be any correlation except that those who suffer with poor sleep and low mood may experience more severe hot flushes.

In general, symptoms tend to get worse as you approach full menopause, which is defined by NICE as a woman not having a period for at least twelve months and not using hormonal contraception.[31]

Athletic performance

If we think research is limited in female athletes, try finding research in perimenopausal and postmenopausal athletes. Until recently, most female athletes would retire from their sporting careers in their mid- to late thirties. While this may still be the case in several sports and at an elite level, more and more women are continuing to compete well into their forties, fifties and sixties. Age-group triathlon, masters running events and the rise of ultra-endurance events, where being an older female may even be an advantage, all encourage participation.

To date, there are no studies that look specifically at athletic performance in this population group, but there is good evidence to back up regular exercise as a way to mitigate against some of the more unpleasant aspects of going through the menopause, including hot flushes, as well as for healthy ageing. [32]

Clinical observation of menopausal athletes I have worked with suggests some of the most common concerns women have relate to increased fatigue, less adaptation from training load and changes to body composition. Additional well-known side effects of the reduction in oestrogen that occurs around the menopause are a reduction in bone density and muscle mass. A varied, nutrient-dense diet with particular focus on sufficient calcium and vitamin D, combined with regular aerobic and resistance exercise, will help to counteract these effects.

BONE HEALTH

Bone density is something that naturally declines with age but accelerates when oestrogen (and testosterone) levels start to diminish. However, this does not mean all is lost. There are several ways you can minimise the loss and also try to improve bone density, even when levels have previously been low.

Ensuring sufficient energy in the body is one important feature, but then the type and frequency of training has a huge influence.

A 2011 study found that: 'Bones become strong when the muscles attached to them become strong. Bone changes are slow, much slower than strength changes. If high-load and low-rep routines of compound exercises are used, these stimulate muscle development around the hips, spine and arms, building bone strength in those vulnerable areas and throughout the body. Even if the [bone density] is not improved, as measured by [DXA] scan, resistance training with adequate intensity will dramatically lower the lifetime fracture risk'.[33]

From the science it is apparent that the maximum load, not the frequency, is most relevant in improving bone density, thus a small number of loading cycles works best.

The bone in the lumbar spine is known as trabecular bone and is directly influenced by nutritional and hormonal status. It is also the type of bone that responds and remodels more rapidly than the cortical bones of the hips

and wrists. It can take four to six months or more for the bone to remodel under the best conditions, and the measurable effects of exercise may only be apparent years later, which is why starting a resistance programme early will have the best benefits and outcome.

Alongside exercise, it is equally important to ensure adequate intakes of calcium – the Recommended Dietary Allowance (RDA) in the UK is 1,000 milligrams per day in this population – and sufficient amounts of vitamin D, which will need to be supplemented.

The best sources of calcium include dairy, soya-based products and oily fish.

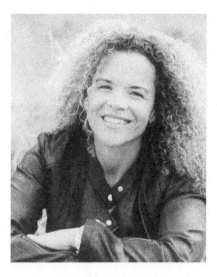

SABRINA'S STORY

I met Sabrina several years ago. She came to me for nutritional advice to support her running. Over the years we have stayed in touch, and we now have the same coach. More recently I have been supporting Sabrina with her charity, Black Trail Runners, encouraging more diversity on the trails.

It's been one of the toughest things I have experienced, continuing to train, to finish races and challenges that I set myself – challenges which seemed so achievable – now I am in perimenopause.

I think that the areas where I have really felt the effects of my hormone levels shifting have been in sleep, recovery and mental focus/resilience.

For many months, before I started on hormone replacement therapy, I struggled to sleep due to night sweats. I would wake up wet all over with a burning heat emanating from my body. I didn't understand what was happening to me. Was I overtrained? Was there something else at play? My bedroom turned into a place of sleepless nights where I would toss, turn and be anxiety-ridden.

My inability to log – on the wearable device sleep tracker I use – the eight hours' sleep that I had been used to started affecting me. As each month went on and my sleep quality got worse, the results of my training in turn became more unpredictable.

I am someone who sets early morning alarms, but I didn't need an alarm at that point as I was already wide awake from the previous evening. Me being tired, dog tired, all day long impacted on my ability to recover appropriately. Every run I went into felt like a slog.

A form of exercise that I have used for years to help me manage my mental health started to negatively impact my mind. 'Why can't I go faster?' 'Why am I so tired?' 'Why do I feel so beaten up all the time?' 'Why is my body working against me?'

Recovery felt like it was taking longer. The techniques and nutrition that once used to help me stay on top of things didn't seem to be giving me what I needed any more.

My resilience, my mental toughness, also started to suffer. I pride myself on being a 'go hard or go home' type of amateur athlete. 'We can do hard things,' I repeat. But easy things – things within my training which I would have flown through years earlier – became super hard. My problem was that I was still assessing myself, my ability, on the athlete that I had been, rather than who I was now. It made me unhappy, it made me feel like an imposter, it fed my depression. My body was changing but, as I didn't really understand the impact on the training cycle, I felt blind.

I asked for advice online and picked up a book by a female doctor, Stacy Sims, and that helped me a lot. It helped me understand what was happening to my body and, due to my cycle, what training might be better for me on different weeks. It also told me – in black and white – that I was not ingesting anywhere near enough protein for recovery. What I thought was a lot was in fact less than half of what I should be looking to consume.

I also went and spoke to my doctor – explained my symptoms, my family history, the fact that the females within my family have all experienced the menopause early. My doctor started me on HRT. I have been on it for six months and feel so much better.

....

PROFESSIONAL OPINION

It is clear that this menopause transition phase of life is challenging. It hits most women hard, but while there is definitely a benefit to having been previously active, the impact it has on fatigue levels, mood and performance can leave you with a real loss of identity.

This period of life can start as early as your late thirties, so many women may not be aware of what is happening to them. Blood tests are important as they will identify changes to hormones and rule out any other concerns such as RED-S or overtraining in those women who are very active.

Sabrina is a case example of how little information there is out there and the importance of education, especially for those of us who want to continue to perform at our premenopause level. My advice is to always go into your GP appointment with as much information as you can get. Remember that being very physically active, while desirable, is also still the minority, and thus GPs may not always be aware of the impact this time of life can have on our performance and, thus, quality of life.

As Sabrina has found, by restoring her declining levels of HRT and modifying her diet, she has been able to maintain her premenopause training load.

....

We can see that regular exercise is recommended for all women going through the perimenopause and postmenopause to mitigate the symptoms and longer-term health consequences.

However, what about when you already have a high training load prior to perimenopause and postmenopause?

As we have previously seen, research in this group of women who partake in regular moderate to heavy training load is limited. Indeed, the postmenopausal women from our survey and those I have worked with in clinic all report noticing changes and a decline in their performance. Mostly this was related to increased fatigue, but also poor recovery between sessions and an inability to maintain previous pace/intensity.

HRT: THE LOW-DOWN

HRT, Hormone Replacement Therapy, is the most effective treatment for improving menopausal symptoms and protecting bone health. Even with this knowledge, there is still a lot of reluctance from many women to take HRT. Unfortunately, this is due to the negative press associated with the Women's Health Initiative study, 2002, which incidentally has since been shown to be flawed. It looked at older women, over sixty, who were given a type of HRT that is no longer used but caused much scaremongering. In general, starting HRT when you are under sixty has huge benefits to your quality of life and health.

HRT consists of replacing the hormones that have declined through menopause, namely oestrogen. It is suggested that ideally this should be transdermal, so through the skin via a patch or gel. For those women who still have their uterus, so they have not had a hysterectomy, they should also take progesterone orally or with the Mirena coil to protect the uterine lining. There are now some variations of HRT available that combine both oestrogen and progesterone in one patch. It is not a one-size-fits-all treatment and it may take a few months to work out what dose is best for you.

Some women worry about the risk of breast cancer with HRT. There is little or no change in the risk of breast cancer if you take oestrogen-only HRT.

Combined HRT can be associated with a small increase in the risk of breast cancer, but talk to your medical practitioner about your concerns.

For those of us who are very active before the menopause, HRT can be a great way to maintain performance, while also benefitting health and actually maintaining and encouraging the deposition of lean muscle mass.

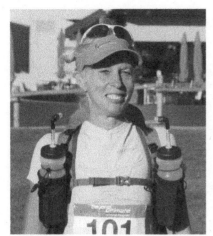

MIMI'S STORY

Mimi contacted me several years ago ahead of her attempt to run across America. We have stayed in touch ever since and I have followed her experience of menopause and performance on social media.

© Martin Paldan

For the past twenty-plus years I have specialised in running long-distance races all over the world. There were many occasions when racing over several days was made tougher when I had my period. Now at the age of fifty-nine, having had no periods for nine years has been incredibly liberating, not just with everyday life but while racing as well; it's the other things my body went through during the menopause I found more of a hindrance and some of the symptoms I had surprised me.

Menopausal symptoms for me began at around forty-seven with the night sweats. I paid very little attention to them at first as they weren't too bad and would disappear quite quickly. Often after big races when I had put my body through a huge amount of pressure I would suffer with night sweats for two or three days, so the night sweats that I was experiencing didn't seem quite as bad.

Roll on eighteen months and the sweats became so severe that I had to go to bed with a couple of towels beside me in preparation for the drenching that would happen during the night.

Having night sweats made me feel pretty revolting, hot, sweaty, smelly and very unattractive. When they happened, all I wanted to do was strip off my clothes and run around outside to cool down (can you imagine the looks I would have got?!); at night I would stick my legs out of the bed until the heat became so intense that the duvet got thrown off. It was a horrid cycle of sweating profusely, then feeling chilled and sticky.

The night sweats meant that my sleep pattern changed. Usually I slept very well, getting around eight hours' sleep, but now I was waking up every couple of hours, which began seriously impacting my training as I woke up feeling tired. Usually I would leap out of bed and head out to train; now I craved an extra few minutes in bed.

Gradually, I began to experience hot flushes during the day; at first they were manageable, but over time they became increasingly worse. Sweat would pour down my chest and face, making me feel incredibly self-conscious and quite honestly pretty disgusting. I could cope with feeling hot, but the combination of hot and sweating began to make me feel extremely embarrassed. I remember going to a meeting in London on a hot day; as I began to talk I could feel the heat rising in me and the sweat began to trickle down my face and chest but I carried on talking. I felt so hot that eventually I grabbed a piece of paper and started fanning myself. One of the men in the meeting very kindly asked if I would like the window open – I thanked him and said the window was already open but not to worry – it was just my time of life! I wasn't embarrassed; he felt slightly uncomfortable.

The day flushes were happening during my runs, which was tough. I had read somewhere that running could help reduce hot flushes. Not in my case. They felt very different from being hot and sweaty from your training session; these flushes would make my whole body feel as though it was overheating, causing me to slow down or have to stop in order to try and cool down; once they had gone, I could continue the run. I always ran in the mornings as this was my preferred time to train, which for menopausal women was supposed to have been the best time, but even this didn't seem to help.

To alleviate the symptoms, I tried various herbal remedies recommended by friends that had worked for them, but nothing seemed to work.

Just before my fiftieth birthday in 2012 I had my last period. I had no idea this was going to happen, as my periods had been pretty regular and I hadn't noticed any change in their intensity or duration.

A couple of months after my last period I set a new world record for running the length of Ireland and had successes in other races, but I was noticing that training/running was becoming more difficult. My legs would begin to ache during my long runs – something I had never experienced before. In a few events the discomfort was incredibly intense: mostly my thighs (on both legs), which would then radiate upwards, impacting my hips; every step I took jarred. I didn't understand why this was happening as I wasn't injured, and when I stopped running my legs felt fine after about thirty minutes. My training had been the same as it had always been and I was used to running long, so it was a complete mystery as to why this was happening.

I went to chat to my doctor about a few of my symptoms, to be told that it was an 'age thing'. I have to admit I came away feeling incredibly deflated and astounded that a doctor, especially a female doctor, should say such a thing.

I noticed a few other things, but these weren't running-related. On the positive side, my sleep pattern had returned to normal, but I continued to feel lethargic. It felt as though my body wasn't working to its full capacity. I spent the day in a sort of fuzzy state, almost as though I was on a drug that was trying to make me sleepy.

I understood that the night sweats and hot flushes were related to the menopause, but I put the other symptoms down to the ageing process, as I had never heard them discussed as menopausal symptoms.

HRT was something that I had wanted to avoid because of the information that had been in the press a few years previously saying it could cause cancer, but I was really struggling; I didn't feel I was in control of my body and was really struggling with my running, which was beginning to feel like a chore rather than something I loved and wanted to do.

Eventually, I had to do something about my situation and went to discuss it with my doctor (a different one!). Together we opted for the pill version of HRT as the one that would best suit me (there are several other options available).

My main concern was weight gain. I had never been able to take the contraceptive pill as it simply sent my hormones all over the place, plus having had an eating disorder, putting on weight was still something I didn't want to do. After several weeks of taking the HRT, I noticed that the night sweats/hot flushes were improving, until eventually they mostly disappeared and there was no weight gain (I don't weigh myself, so went by my clothes). The lethargy and leg aches went and I noticed that my intolerance of things and people improved. I felt as though my normal self was beginning to reappear.

I stayed on the HRT for a few years, having regular check-ups, but unfortunately the brand of HRT I was taking was stopped. The doctor told me not to worry – they would put me on another brand of the same dosage. Unfortunately, I have had to go through several strengths and brands of HRT to find another one that worked. During this time, the hot flushes came back, I became increasingly intolerant of even the smallest thing, the lethargy returned, making going out for training sessions a real effort. I was back to square one.

After several trips to the doctor's surgery I was eventually put on an HRT pill that worked. I'm feeling back to my old self once more. It's been hard at times to stay positive, but it's wonderful to once more feel that my body is where it should be – happy!

....

PROFESSIONAL OPINION

Once again, it is clear from Mimi's story that the information out there regarding the menopause in general is poor, let alone if you are someone who has always been physically active. The lack of education around HRT, the different options and the misinformation regarding the potential side effects all need to improve to ensure women feel supported during this huge time of change.

While it took Mimi a while, it is clear that HRT has not only improved her quality of life, but also has a significant impact on maintaining her performance.

....

Nutrition and training

Nutritionally, ensuring a good mix of nutrient-dense foods, wholegrains, fruit and vegetables, legumes, lean choices of protein, dairy and/or soya will help to meet all macro- and micronutrient requirements. In addition, this way of eating will support a diverse and healthy gut microbiome. Declining hormone levels can have a negative impact on digestion and gut health. As discussed earlier, regular moderate-intensity exercise and a varied diet which meets energy availability supports a healthy gut biome and has been shown to result in positive responses in performance, but also negates the impact on digestion due to falling hormone levels.

Summary of key points

The transition through to menopause can be a challenging time. Fluctuating hormones result in a barrage of symptoms of varying severity, which can last for as long as a decade. While this is an area that is of real interest, research is limited, especially in the athlete population. However, with many women pursuing their sports later into life, understanding strategies and practices that can support both health and performance is paramount.

Changes to body composition seems to be one of the key driving forces to change nutritional practices, with lower-carbohydrate diets being favoured. We have already seen how low-carbohydrate diets may impact performance. Thus, while it may seem like an appropriate option, it has to be weighed against the potential negative impacts on both physical and psychological health, especially in light of the increased fatigue experienced by women at this stage. Postmenopausal women, particularly those maintaining higher levels of physical activity, may benefit from higher intakes of carbohydrate due to the loss of oestrogen that encourages fat oxidation, sparing carbohydrate.

CHAPTER 8

The Masters Athlete

Introduction

We live in a world of increasingly ageing populations, with those over sixty-five now outnumbering those under five.[34] Regular physical activity, supported by a good diet, is a hugely important part of healthy ageing, protecting against many of the common causes of morbidity and mortality caused by a sedentary lifestyle and exacerbated by older age. Staying physically active also improves mental health and well-being, facilitates social contact, and reduces the risk of falls and fractures in older people.

When it comes to athletics competitions, a masters athlete is anyone above the age of thirty-five, but in reality, the greatest age-related changes happen to us a little later than that. As we reach older ages, the effects reach right across our physiology, including reduced muscle mass and strength, reduced bone density, increased fat mass, and decreased glucose metabolism and cardiovascular function. Metabolic rate changes little between the ages of twenty and sixty, after which it too begins its inexorable decline.

Training for healthy, active ageing

The good news is that appropriate training and diet can at least reduce the severity of many of these changes. Many recreational athletes continue to perform well into their forties and fifties, often outperforming younger participants in events of a longer duration.

Declines in muscle mass are directly linked with physical activity, with sedentary, inactive peers experiencing a more rapid decline. Resistance training seems to be pivotal in maintaining mass in this population, so the addition of two to three sessions a week on top of normal training can reap huge benefits.

Most studies on training effects in this population have been done on male athletes and, while it has been shown that 30% of men over the age of fifty have some element of testosterone deficiency, in most males, testosterone levels stay stable, and this may also have a protective effect in preventing losses in muscle mass in those individuals who remain active. This potential performance-enhancing role of testosterone is one of the reasons it is on the banned list within sport. Thus, those men who do have a testosterone deficiency should be encouraged to seek medical advice.

Women, as we know, will start to see declining levels of oestrogen from around forty years onwards. Studies that have looked at women of this age group have demonstrated that those women who choose not to take hormone replacement therapy are most likely to see a downward trend in their body composition, cardiac output and overall physical performance. Indeed, it is the advance in HRT, especially the transdermal option, that has allowed so many women to not only have a better quality of life but also maintain the physical performance throughout their lifetime.

Bone density decreases as testosterone and oestrogen start to diminish. Sarcopenia (the progressive and generalised loss of skeletal muscle mass and strength) affects both sexes during the ageing process, particularly in the absence of a good diet. A UK Biobank study in 2021 found that '5,950 (8%) of the 74,293 women and 4,075 (5.1%) of the 80,136 men were pre-sarcopenic or sarcopenic. Overall, compared with non-sarcopenic individuals, both men and women with pre-sarcopenia or sarcopenia were older, more likely to currently smoke, use H2 blockers and/or corticosteroids, and report never drinking alcohol. They had lower levels of physical activity and reported a lower intake of protein and calcium.'[35]

When it comes to looking at training specifically, we have already identified that resistance training is paramount for maintaining muscle mass and thus helping to slow physical declines in strength and performance. An interesting study from the US looked at three different training groups of male participants over a period of twenty-two years.[36] The first group of runners trained strenuously through this study period; the second group maintained their running but at a more relaxed, steady pace; and the third group became sedentary. All participants were in their mid- to late forties when they were retested.

Those who were in the sedentary group exhibited characteristic declines in fitness, including a 15%-per-decade loss of aerobic capacity, a twelve-beat-per-minute reduction in maximal heart rate, a waning of running efficiency and a significant shortening of stride length.

Those in the easy running group lost about 9% of aerobic capacity per decade, just under the expected 10–15%.

Those who continued training at a high level had no significant loss of Vo2 max, maximal heart rate, running economy or stride length, even though they had matured from their mid-twenties into their late forties.

The researchers concluded that, 'If you stay highly motivated and injury-free and continue training at a decent intensity during your forties and fifties, you just don't lose very much.'

Fuelling for healthy, active ageing

There is no question that an athlete, regardless of sporting discipline, can continue to train and perform well into their older years. With the right approach to training, and sufficient recovery, meaning more rest days than previously, optimal performance and outcome can be maintained. However, irrespective of the age of the athlete, appropriate nutrition is integral to supporting and encouraging adaptation from training.

To a certain degree, when it comes to an optimal diet to support both health and physical activity, very little changes. Staying physically active and eating a well-balanced supportive diet is the best way to slow many of the declines associated with getting older. Meeting energy requirements and adjusting according to activity level is still critical to ensure optimal health, progression and performance. Similarly, carbohydrate requirements remain the same as discussed in chapter 1 of this book and, once again, are dependent on training load. As a side note, with the current recommendations for masters athletes to maintain a certain level of high-intensity training, carbohydrate availability – particularly around these training sessions – is going to be paramount to drive the hormonal cascade necessary to support adaptation. Particular attention should be paid to rest days for older athletes, as recovery can take longer, but good energy availability and nutrition should be maintained on rest days to support this recovery. It can take up to seventy-two hours for recovery after high-intensity efforts or long endurance sessions, so paying attention to nutrition during these rest periods is equally as important as fuelling for training.

As well as maintaining physical activity and incorporating more resistance training, ensuring that there is enough protein in the diet will also help to prevent the usual decline in muscle mass associated with this population. Studies have shown that masters athletes should aim for a minimum of 1.2 grams of protein per kilogram of body weight per day, but are more likely to need up to 1.6 grams per kilogram of body weight per day. This is higher than younger athletes and is related to a decline in muscle protein synthesis, thus more protein availability is required to increase uptake. Those who consume good amounts of protein have been shown to maintain 40% more muscle mass than those who have low intake of protein. In addition to the overall protein intake, a good distribution through the day seems to improve overall retention and encourage the adaptive responses. The recommendations are 0.4 grams per kilogram of body weight per meal as well as in the immediate post-exercise phase and later in the evening before bed. This works out at 28 grams of protein in a 70-kilogram athlete. Furthermore, the quality of protein seems to be equally as important, and whole protein sources are recommended where possible. This includes eggs, milk, Greek yoghurt, meat, poultry and fish. Those who follow a plant-based diet will need to be mindful that they consume the right variety of foods throughout the day to ensure that their amino acid requirements are being met, as discussed in part 1.

We know that including n-3 (omega-3) fatty acids benefits the athlete diet. Recent research suggests that there may be further advantages in male older athletes as n-3 fatty acids are associated with an increase in the rate of muscle protein synthesis, but data is limited and further studies are required. However, we know there are general health benefits to including n-3 fatty acids in the diet. Thus, ensuring a weekly intake of oily fish or using a regular supplement may be considered.

As with all athletes, micronutrients will need to be individually monitored, but special care should be taken with vitamin D. As we get older, the skin's capacity to produce vitamin D from sunlight deteriorates.

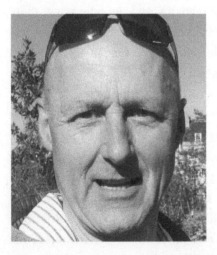

PAUL'S STORY

I met Paul when I joined Team Bath Athletics Club. We were often in the same training group and attended the same races. Not only is Paul great fun to be around but, due to his disposition, he is also a huge inspiration.

I came to proper running relatively late having been a keen amateur footballer for most of my sporting life. I decided at the age of forty-eight, having broken yet another bone, to hang my boots up and look for other physical challenges. This came in the form of local half-marathon races, which I found enjoyably challenging and satisfying. I ran my first marathon in my fiftieth year in Edinburgh and managed a reasonable three hours sixteen minutes for an 'old bloke'.

'Join a running club' was the advice from friends, and after some research I chose Team Bath AC as it was close to home and based at the prestigious University of Bath Sports Training Village.

I loved running and racing with other enthusiastic and friendly athletes, quickly becoming absorbed into the world of athletics, and endurance running in particular.

My road event was the marathon, and my proudest moment and 'fifteen minutes of fame' was completing the World Majors Marathon Series (London, Berlin, Boston, Chicago, New York and Tokyo) in 2014. My average time of three hours twenty minutes, although not the fastest, was still okay for an ever-maturing athlete. I also enjoyed cross-country racing, partly due to it being a team event, but mainly because of the mud!

Avoiding injury and burnout is the secret to successful endurance running. Unfortunately, at the age of sixty my arthritic left hip required resurfacing joint replacement surgery (probably a consequence of far too much football in my younger years!). Perhaps my marathon and athletic days were at an end? This all coincided with my planned retirement from a busy but rewarding career as a hospital consultant. I now had the time and energy to rehabilitate from my hip surgery as well as pursuing a long-term ambition to gain my higher UK Athletics Coaching qualifications alongside further practical training in Strength and Conditioning. Although I had to cut down on my running, I maintained my aerobic fitness and love of exercise through more road cycling, and swimming.

So where am I at today? My hip operation has been a brilliant success to date and I am back doing more running miles and the occasional low-key competition. Although I still enjoy cycling and swimming, they don't quite provide the same happiness as running wild over the hills and trails.

I enjoy my role as senior endurance running coach with Team Bath AC and endeavour to share my drive, knowledge and passion with others. We have many excellent masters athletes at the club and I find the challenge of helping them to be the 'best they can be' very rewarding. It is amazing what can be achieved through combining human endeavour with smart training and conditioning.

For myself, I am an acknowledged 'exercise junkie', whether it's outside via the road and trail or inside in the gym and swimming pool. I love the physical challenge and mental buzz of exercise. I am a staunch advocate of strength and conditioning in order to enable the body to be as resilient and co-ordinated as possible. High-Intensity Interval Training in its various forms provides extra gain and has been shown to have proven health benefits. I also strongly recommend and practise a 'heavy weights session' every seven to fourteen days in an effort to maintain muscle strength and improve neuro-muscular recruitment. For strength, muscle activation, range of movement, enhanced breathing and mindfulness, the disciplines of Pilates and yoga provide a robust adjunct to my training which I encourage all to explore.

Together with my training and exercise, I also ensure that I have access to a personal trainer, physiotherapist, nutritionist and sports masseur alongside the constant friendship of my fellow athletes.

Sport and physical exercise have been my lifelong companions and continue to be. They bring me great joy, emotion and well-being.

PROFESSIONAL OPINION

Paul's account and experience fit in line with the recommendations that are encouraged for older/masters athletes, and it is great to see that the science pays off, regardless of your training level. As someone who was always very active, the best thing Paul has done is to maintain his training load. While he may mix it up these days, he includes the essential resistance training and interval work that has most definitely been effective. At sixty-six years of age, Paul shows no sign of slowing down, but it's great that he equally appreciates the importance of nutrition and rest.

Summary of key points

Staying physically active and eating well are the best ways to reduce the loss of bone and muscle mass, along with other factors associated with ageing, thus mitigating the decline in performance and changes to body composition.

While an older athlete should include more overall rest in their training schedule, incorporating some higher-intensity sessions, as well as resistance training two or three times a week, is paramount in maintaining optimal performance.

Nutritionally, ensuring energy requirements are being met, especially carbohydrate availability, around high intensity or long endurance sessions is key.

Ensuring regular intakes of 25–40 grams of good-quality protein, three to five times throughout the day, helps to ensure muscle adaptation.

Always ensure a good recovery choice post-training that contains both carbohydrate and protein. Recovery can take a little longer in older athletes, so being mindful of nutrition at this stage is necessary to allow for adequate recovery prior to your next session. Good options include milkshakes, bagels and eggs, jacket potato and tuna, or Greek yoghurt and granola.

Consider taking a daily supplement of vitamin D during the winter months, especially in the northern hemisphere.

CHAPTER 9

The Individual Athlete

Introduction

What do I mean by the individual athlete?

From its traditionally white, male, middle-class, able-bodied roots, recreational sport in the UK is slowly becoming more diverse, inclusive and accepting. Some sports are doing this better than others, but there is still so much more to do. The real aim of this chapter is to highlight the importance of being your own athlete. Regardless of race, genetics, gender, age, socio-economic status, or even what the evidence does or doesn't say, it's about championing those of you who may not always be seen or heard, and encouraging you to participate in sport for the joy it brings you.

When I think about my own relationship and journey with sport, it hasn't been straightforward. As someone who comes from a minority background, sport was not really something that was hugely encouraged over academia. That said, I have definitely been fortunate and privileged that a diversity of sport has always been available to me. In more recent years, I have had to learn how to maintain my love of running while also managing sarcoidosis, an autoimmune lung condition. While it would be easy to focus on what it feels like to be a diverse athlete, it is not only those of us from minority backgrounds who are overlooked in sport. So much of the information and evidence available is focused on highly trained male athletes from Western cultures and most of the opportunity goes to those who are affluent. In the previous two chapters we have already looked at two population groups that are generally off the radar – although, again, change is happening.

But what about those who are not able-bodied? Or who don't have access or financial means to participate in sport? What about those who have chronic health conditions such as autoimmune or depression, or who are in remission from a serious illness such as cancer?

How do all these groups navigate what to eat, how to train and how to maintain optimal performance?

Eating behaviours and nutritional requirements

One of the many pleasures of living in a country with such a dense diversity in cultural backgrounds is the opportunity to taste new food flavours and dishes. Indeed, look at most cities in the UK and the abundance of choice is a real privilege – Lebanese, Indian, Vietnamese, French and Caribbean, to name but a few.

When working with people from different backgrounds, whether they are athletes or not, I always make sure that I have done my research on their traditional diets. If we are going to encourage people to eat well, then it is also important to ensure that we provide them with choices that they can relate to, as it means they are most likely going to comply and engage. So while we know that this group of individual athletes will still need to maintain good carbohydrate availability around their training, it is important to ensure that we provide options that are acceptable to them.

This also highlights another really important point, which is that while the avoidance of certain foods is often encouraged prior to sporting events and competition, if these foods usually make up a high percentage of the diet, removing them may be more problematic and result in a lower energy intake, having a negative effect on performance. One example would be the high composition of beans and lentils in Indian diets. The sports-nutrition recommendations state that high-fibre foods should be avoided twenty-four to forty-eight hours prior to competition, but we have to appreciate that an Indian athlete will have the gut microbiome that means they are able to tolerate and digest these foods better than non-Indian athletes (head back to chapter 1 to read more on the gut microbiome).

Similarly, other cultures may put a lot of importance on red meat; while this will be great for their iron intake and stores, it may also mean that they displace this for carbohydrate-based foods which will help their performance. In the same context, other cultures may be devoid of certain foods, meaning they tend to be at a higher risk of nutritional deficiencies.

What about if your diet is limited due to a chronic health condition, such as coeliac?

Coeliac disease is an autoimmune condition, meaning the body's immune system attacks and destroys healthy body tissue in error.

Gluten is the protein found within wheat and related grains, including barley and rye. It is therefore found in foods such as bread, pasta and cereals, but also in sausages and beer. For most individuals, gluten does not pose a problem. The body has the ability to break it down, as with other proteins, absorb it and utilise it as necessary. However, for those individuals who are diagnosed with coeliac disease, gluten needs to be avoided, as consumption of it affects the small intestine, causing it to become damaged and unable to absorb vital nutrients such as calcium, iron and energy from food. The symptoms are usually weight loss, extreme fatigue due to iron deficiency, bloating and very frequent bowel movements. Due to an inability to absorb calcium, those who have coeliac disease may also be at an increased risk of osteoporosis, which makes your bones weak, putting you at a greater risk of fractures and breaks if you fall.

Coeliac disease is usually confirmed by taking blood tests and gut biopsies. The individual will then be put on a strict gluten-free diet, which they will need to comply with for life.

Similarly, a small percentage of individuals suffer from wheat allergy. Unlike the symptoms for coeliac disease, wheat allergy tends to affect the skin but can also be linked with some gastrointestinal symptoms; the difference being that there are no structural changes that are detrimental to absorption as occurs in coeliac disease. There is usually an immediate allergic reaction that causes itchy skin and itchy eyes, and there may even be swelling of both eyes and throat. A wheat allergy is usually diagnosed by skin-prick testing, and the individual will need to remove all wheat from their diet.

So in these situations and other scenarios where certain food groups have to be avoided due to intolerances, allergies or general disagreement with the body, more care will need to be taken in ensuring that nutritional needs for training can be met, particularly carbohydrate where wheat and gluten are an issue, and in recovery choices where lactose or dairy is problematic. While living with a chronic illness and participating in sport is possible, it will take a bit more planning and knowledge around what to choose. It may be a case of trial and error until you find the approach that works for you.

It's not just cultural differences and chronic illness that we have to consider when contemplating nutritional needs and preferences. The number of athletes participating in para- and disability sport is increasing. Around 4,300 athletes participated in the 2016 Summer Paralympics in Rio, and this increased slightly to just over 4,400 athletes in Tokyo in 2021.

In the lead-up to Rio 2016, I worked in two disability sports: GB wheelchair basketball and GB wheelchair fencing. One of the biggest challenges I faced was the lack of scientific studies available to help understand nutritional requirements. As in all sports, there was so much to consider from training age and education around nutritional needs and training load, but also the specific disability and what was required for optimal performance. For example, an athlete with spinal-cord injury has very different needs from an athlete with cerebral palsy. To date, data relating to nutritional requirements in disability athletes is scant, but one review in 2018 looked at energy and nutrient issues in athletes with spinal-cord injuries.[37] The researchers stated upfront that due to the limited studies available in this population group, both sedentary individuals and para-athletes with spinal cord injuries were included. Even with this diversity in spinal-cord individuals, which no doubt will have skewed the results, the general conclusion was that more studies were required; but it was clear that athletes with spinal-cord injuries were at high risk of low energy availability and micronutrient deficiencies. Specifically, when compared with able-bodied athletes' intakes of carbohydrate grams per kilogram of body weight, intakes were significantly lower, while protein consumption was similar.

One thing is clear: there is a lot more to consider when working with disability athletes. The impact their disability and related clinical features may have on metabolism sweat rates, and thus fluid losses, and the cost of involuntary movement associated with some disabilities, is still largely unknown. Care must be taken to ensure that these individual athletes do not feel pressure to conform to body ideals that are commonly associated with athletes and performance, as they may not be realistically achievable. And, finally, there needs to be some understanding and respect for food preferences, beliefs and upbringing, while equally avoiding nutritional deficiencies.

During my experience, I used what research data was available while also responding to the athlete in front of me, thus providing a very individualised approach. I tailored advice based on my vast clinical and sports-nutrition knowledge and experience, as well as extrapolating from any research that was available. I monitored progress by regularly talking to both the individual athlete and coach, and then amended as needed.

That said, this is central to my practice, regardless of who I work with, and I guess highlights the importance of individuals, regardless of ethnicity, sporting ability or level, finding a dietary and training approach that works for them. There will always be recommendations and preferences, but even if the science backs a particular way of eating, it doesn't always mean it is relevant to you.

Thus, when it comes to nutritional practices specifically, until we have more robust studies on the differences between athletes from different backgrounds and their nutritional requirements, the key messaging probably needs to be the same, ensuring sufficient energy availability, particular carbohydrate availability around training and optimal recovery strategies. This may prove challenging in some circumstances. For example, we know that clinical depression can suppress your appetite, but we also know that gentle to moderate movement and being outdoors has significant benefits for mental health. This situation also highlights the difference between movement, exercise and training. For some of us, just moving is enough to support our mental well-being and health. These individuals will benefit from making nutrient-dense choices, but the first step may be just getting them to be more active. When we look at exercise, this may be about staying fit, losing additional weight to improve health metrics, being social and just enjoying participating in sport. Training is more focused – there is usually a performance outcome, whether that is speed, body composition or a distance to accomplish. In this situation, it is important to take more care about the timing of nutrition and ensuring sufficient energy.

Summary of key points

From the data that is available, it is clear there is still a lot of work to be done in order to achieve equal representation across sport and sports coaching. Some of this is about the opportunities available and changing messages to avoid discrimination, but some of this is also about educating different cultures and population groups of the benefits of participation in sport and making these scenarios available and affordable.

Some organisations are taking this into their own hands. Companies like Ultra X have made a pledge to encourage more diversity at their races, and earlier this year I took part in one of them where I was so heartened by the fact that there was a much bigger percentage of BAME runners present across all the distances. Trail Running Nepal is another such company that I have had the pleasure of working alongside and taking part in their races. They ensure they provide free places to local Nepalese runners in all their races, but also help to get them out to some of the bigger, more mainstream mountain-running events.

Brands are also sitting up and taking notice. Personally, I have been approached by many sports brands in recent years, all wanting to not just highlight my professional voice but also promote the fact that I take part in sport to encourage others to see that it is possible and should not be stigmatised. Similarly, I have noticed more and more individuals who have chronic conditions such as cystic fibrosis, inflammatory bowel disease and type 1 diabetes talking about the benefits of exercise on their conditions and demonstrating that it is not only possible, but you can also be competitive if you want.

Organisations like Black Trail Runners and TrailFam are all working towards making sports – and running specifically – acceptable and available to all, while also generating some very cool role models.

Regardless of your situation, remember there is a dietary and training approach that will work for you, and this may also need to change as time goes on. I know with my sarcoidosis, there are times when I have to pull back training considerably. I often change things up, focusing on yoga and more resistance training. On the whole I'm guided by my appetite, but also keep in mind the nutritional requirements for this type of exercise. Remember, there will always be recommendations and preferences, but even if the science backs a particular way of eating, it doesn't always mean it is relevant to you or your present situation.

Before I end this chapter, I want to highlight that the above is just an introduction to this topic around 'the individual athlete' and I've just addressed the tip of the iceberg on this subject.

I want to thank Vertebrate for encouraging me to speak out and discuss these athlete groups that are under-represented and so often overlooked. My key observations are that a lot more research is necessary, but hopefully even this short chapter will start to encourage a more open dialogue.

CHAPTER 10

Over to You

As stated right at the start of this book, the aim here is not to tell you what to do. I wanted to provide you with all the research and science in a palatable format so that you, as individuals, can make an informed choice about what is the best nutritional approach for you.

As we have seen, there is a lot to consider and many influences. It is not as simple as following your athlete aspiration; it is clear that focusing on one outcome alone can potentially lead to several other scenarios that are not as favourable.

With the rise in popularity of social media as a means of communication and influence, social comparison and human behaviour, it is easy to see why messages around food, training and performance can get so confused.

While there are some great accounts on social media, there are also many accounts that use their own personal anecdotal experience in 'educating' the masses. Poor understanding and interpretation of the science, and cherry-picking evidence to support messages, even when the population group or study model is not appropriate, all contribute to the lack of clarity and, in some cases, dysfunctional behaviours with long-lasting health and performance consequences.

Equally, we cannot forget the role of human behaviour. Humans are complex and human behaviour is unpredictable. While our brains are highly sophisticated organs, psychologists have reported that social media is having a huge impact not only on the structure of our brains but also on our cognition, specifically social cognition affecting our self-concepts and self-esteem.

One example of this is when uncertainty arises. When we think about this logically, it is an inevitable part of life. No one really knows what is coming next. The human brain, especially an anxious one, struggles with gaps – so, when a potential outcome is not known, it will go in search of an answer. This might be through a previous experience, or by filling the gap with a definitive negative. The human brain finds it much easier to accept this than 'I don't know!'

While the individual may be satisfied that they now have an outcome, this not only serves as a false sense of security, but it can also play into a self-fulfilling prophecy.

What do I mean by this?

Let us take the example of an athlete who is getting recurrent injuries. The rational approach would be to consider their training load. However, previous experience has shown them that at this load they can achieve a PB. They do not know what would happen if they introduced more rest days, but the uncertainty of the situation, the 'I don't know' and the potential anxiety causes their brain to assume the worst-case scenario. That is, if they reduce their training load, they will lose fitness and thus impact their performance. This is a limiting belief. It stops the individual from moving into a space of unknown, which will cause them anxiety and discomfort. At the same time, it also provides them with an 'answer'. The more they cycle this belief around, the more it becomes their truth and impacts their behaviour, even though there is no factual evidence that this is the right solution.

Modern society has made us all very outcome-focused, with little thought given to the processes that are required. Many successful elite athletes have reported that their biggest lessons have been learnt from situations that haven't worked out for them, and yet so many of us are fearful of failing.

While many individuals participate in sport for health and well-being, there are also a high percentage of recreational athletes who train hard and take their sport very seriously. These particular recreational athletes tend to be driven and, as we stated earlier, can also become confused by having a perfectionist mindset. The two are very different. Drive and motivation are helpful traits and tend to go hand in hand with a growth mindset. Perfectionism is an impossible task, but the individual is never satisfied, and their pursuit is often futile and results in dysfunctional and unhelpful behaviours.

Perfectionists will often see life as black and white: something is good or bad, there is right and wrong, this will happen or it won't. There is a real sense of permanence in their mindset, and yet we know that nothing in life is permanent or fixed – life is transitional and not linear. Thus, those athletes who navigate life more effectively tend to appreciate they need to often operate in the grey.

The aim of the book is to help you see the potential shades of grey regarding nutrition, training and performance, to help you make the right choice for you. We know that no one size fits all. We have also seen from the numerous case studies that everyone is different. So even when the science tells us one thing, it may not consider different lifestyles, training age, gender, body types and personal preference. Thus, to a certain degree, there is no right or wrong approach. Some nutritional behaviours may create more risk and be less suited to certain individuals. The key is having the full picture, being mindful of the potential risks, so that if symptoms or undesirable situations start to occur, you appreciate where they are coming from and can change appropriately.

With that in mind, let's revisit the four main nutritional approaches and the special considerations to see where care might be needed.

Low-carbohydrate, high-fat

While this has proven to be a very popular approach in many sports, especially climbing and endurance, the science is clear. For individuals who train at different intensities, as you would expect when trying to achieve a specific performance outcome, a low-carbohydrate approach is not suitable as it has been shown to be detrimental to performance and can also impact long-term health.

There are some therapeutic scenarios where this approach has proven successful – for example, for those with certain types of epilepsy, and it can be used in the short term with type 2 diabetes to help reverse the condition. However, it is unlikely that either of these situations are going to involve high-intensity exercise. It is important to note that, even with type 2 diabetes, the intervention is short-term.

We saw very different outcomes from our two case studies, even though both were runners. Holly is female and trains at a very high level, whereas Stephen is male and, although he trains regularly, maybe doesn't include quite the same training load or intensity. We know that women are particularly susceptible to low carbohydrate intakes, as this has a direct effect on their production of the thyroid hormone, T3. Although the same situation occurs in males, it is more sensitive and thus rapid in women, most likely due to one of the many roles oestrogen plays in the female body.

So, is it ever appropriate to go low-carbohydrate?

From a scientific point of view, if you want to maintain performance and ensure adaptation from your training, ditching carbohydrate is not the answer.

Many believe that a low-carbohydrate diet will lead to weight loss. Initially this may occur, but this is due to fluid loss associated with empty muscle glycogen stores, not changes to actual body composition. Indeed, studies looking at weight loss over longer time frames show that there is no significant difference in outcome, regardless of whether you follow a low-carbohydrate, high-fat approach, or a low-fat, moderate-carbohydrate approach. However, the low-fat, moderate-carbohydrate approach is easier to sustain.

This is particularly important to consider in those in menopause transition and postmenopause, who often decide to go low-carbohydrate, high-fat to help with body composition changes associated with declining oestrogen levels. For women who are looking to maintain high levels of intensity and performance, HRT and a diet adequate in energy, carbo-hydrate availability and protein is the best approach. A low-carbohydrate intake will exacerbate fatigue and stress within the body, amplifying symptoms and low mood.

In younger athletes, a low-carbohydrate, high-fat approach would never be indicated or advised, but in older people who may have not previously trained but are taking up physical activity at a low-to-moderate intensity, this approach may be suitable. It is not a necessity, but if it is a way of eating the individual would prefer to follow, then it would be a situation where this is appropriate. I would caveat that with being mindful about the potential risks that were explained in chapter 2. Perhaps a lower-carbohydrate, rather than low-carbohydrate, approach would be more suitable.

We have already spoken about the importance of carbohydrate, particularly wholegrains, fruit and legumes, with regard to the gut biome. These foods not only encourage a diversity of gut flora, but they also aid digestion. Thus, it is not uncommon to become constipated following a low-carbohydrate, high-fat diet. One further undesirable side effect is halitosis or bad breath due to the production of ketones for energy in the absence of glucose.

The final word on low-carbohydrate, high-fat diets: while they have received a huge amount of attention and traction, there are very few scenarios where they are an appropriate and, to a certain degree, safe choice.

Those individuals, like our case study Stephen, who have reported perceived benefits don't need to change, but should be mindful of the potential risks and consequences.

Those who are considering this approach should think clearly about the reason behind their choice. If performance and body composition are central to their decision, then this may not be the most appropriate way of eating.

Plant-based diets

On paper, plant-based diets incorporate many of the components associated with a healthy diet. Wholegrains, legumes and plentiful colours of fruit and vegetables all promote a diverse gut biome, which has positive associations in supporting our immune and mental health. Although many worry about protein intakes, a well-balanced and planned approach means that most individuals should meet their requirements.

That said, one population group that may be at a slight disadvantage is the older athlete. Research has shown that a higher intake of protein in this group is necessary to prevent lean muscle mass losses that are more likely as we age. It is suggested that where possible this should be from whole protein sources that provide all essential amino acids. Plant-based proteins are not complete, and while it is possible to consume a good mix through the day, the higher volume and bulk of food required to hit target requirements may prove problematic. There is some suggestion that the lack of whole protein sources in plant-based diets may be a limiting factor in maintaining strength and thus preventing a decline in performance. This can be avoided, as with our case study, where a more flexible approach is taken and, while Damian follows a predominantly plant-based diet, he ensures he meets his protein requirements to support his training load.

In the same way, the sheer volume of food needed to meet energy requirements through a plant-based diet may result in unintentional but chronic low energy availability. Working with a nutritional professional to help understand nutritional needs and delivery around training load can help to mitigate this risk.

A plant-based approach can be suitable for athletes if time is taken to ensure attention to detail. It is not just macronutrients that need to be considered; micronutrients are just as important, as they are essential for so many biological processes to work effectively. Some micronutrients can be harder to source from a plant-based diet; familiarising yourself with good sources and taking supplements if needed ensures that no deficiencies occur. We addressed the key nutrients in chapter 2.

In general, a plant-based approach can work for athletes, but coaches, sports-science teams, friends and family need to be vigilant with certain types of individuals. These individuals use the label of being 'plant-based' as a means of over-restricting their nutritional intake. It can become an easy way to disguise disordered eating and/or an eating disorder, as there is a 'legitimate' reason to remove food groups. These individuals can be identified as their focus is not ensuring they achieve balance and all the nutrients they require; it is very much about the 'plant-based' label. For example, when I work with an athlete who wants to achieve optimal health and performance, if I say that they should switch almond milk for soya milk as it has more protein, they accept this and have no issue with putting this into play. However, when I'm working with someone who has a more disordered approach, they find excuse after excuse to avoid ensuring their diet is nutrient-dense and appropriate for their activity levels. These individuals are at huge risk of low energy availability and RED-S.

There are several real positives of following a plant-based diet. For individuals who want to improve key health metrics such as reducing cholesterol, improving blood glucose control and encouraging weight maintenance, combining a plant-based approach with regular physical activity – even just starting to walk for up to forty minutes three times a week – can be hugely beneficial.

Athletes and those who are physically very active will need to be more careful to ensure that not only are overall energy requirements met, but special care is taken to incorporate the right foods to meet their protein needs. While they may have to have a bit more of a flexible approach, with careful planning and good education, being totally or at least predominantly plant-based is totally achievable.

Intermittent fasting

IF is predominantly known as a weight-loss approach. You either love it or you hate it. In theory, it makes sense – you limit your window of eating, or you restrict yourself to a very low-calorie intake two days a week, thus creating an energy deficit resulting in weight loss. And yet, when compared with regular calorie-counting weight-loss strategies, there doesn't seem to be any significance between the two options. Fundamentally, they are pretty much one and the same thing – a way of controlling energy intake.

So, are there any benefits?

Scientists have found that for some individuals there is a psychological benefit to having a time frame to work within. It provides structure.

In addition, as there are a few different options available, individuals can find the plan that works best for them. However, on the flip side of this, most people fall off the IF wagon due to the lack of flexibility and the impact it has on their social life. Where traditional calorie-counting means that you can still meet up with friends, even if you are being mindful of your nutritional intake, IF will have its limitation, based on your chosen window for eating.

In the same way, while some people find reducing their eating window to be a helpful aid to curtailing their overall energy intake, others find that breaking the fast is almost like opening the floodgates. Indeed, human physiology supports this. Remember that the human body is biased towards energy balance and prefers to be in a positive energy balance rather than a negative one. So, when a fast is broken, there is a tendency for the body to go in search of food and even eat to excess to stock up for when food once again becomes scarce. This latter point is probably the key contributor to why many people can't sustain an IF approach but also find that, in the long run, it doesn't result in weight loss.

From our own survey, very few athletes chose and maintained IF, with only one of the subjects admitting that it was something he had recently started. Indeed, the data on IF specifically with the athletic/physically very active in mind is limited. Most information comes from looking at those who follow the religious practice of Ramadan, with the results not showing favourable benefits to performance. Our own case study backed this up, explaining how mindful Taz needs to be not to over-stress her system and to manage her fatigue levels. Outside of Ramadan, she sees no benefits to IF.

With all this in mind, it is interesting to observe that the practice of fasted training is still very popular. Some put this down to convenience: they can get up early and go without having to worry about digesting. Others find that they just can't stomach any form of food before any training, while the most common reason is still tied up with performance. Many individuals still believe that fasted training, or 'training low', improves their ability to become 'fat-adapted' – that is, utilise more fat for fuel during physical activity. This was discussed in detail in chapter 2 but, fundamentally, if performance is your goal, then fasted training is not best practice.

IF is used by many, but it is more challenging in those who want to maintain a high training load. For those individuals who legitimately need to lose weight and like a structure to follow, IF may be a good option. To a degree, it takes out the stress of calorie counting, as you are limiting the window of time in which you can consume energy. However, it is important to note that physical activity will need to be managed and most likely completed during the eating window, especially if the goal is changes to body composition and some performance gains.

The only other time that I may use this method specifically with athletes is in those sports where you need to make weight. However, I caveat this with the fact that I would monitor the athlete closely, especially if training load was high. It would only be done for a relatively short period of time – less than two weeks – and training would never come during or immediately after the fast.

To conclude, when it comes to a weight-loss trend, IF has had a lot of attention but, as we saw in chapter 2, research specifically relating to athletes and performance is scant, making it difficult to support.

Weight-loss/Calorie-control approaches

It has often been stated that over half the population will be on a diet at some point in their lives and yet, having an overweight/obese population is still one of the Western world's biggest challenges.

This would suggest that, as such, diets don't work.

Indeed, a 2020 study in the *BMJ* looked at a total of 22,000 subjects who were either categorised as overweight (with a BMI over 25) or obese (BMI over 30) via 122 different weight-loss trials, which focused on the most popular approaches to losing weight. The outcome showed that while in the first six months of all approaches, moderate weight loss, reduced blood pressure and cardiovascular risks were observed, by twelve months none of this had been sustained.[38]

As we discussed in chapter 2, the human body doesn't like being in a deficit, but also, when an individual loses weight, especially as this will be a combination of both body fat and lean muscle mass, metabolic rate decreases. This means that intakes need to keep being reduced to maintain weight loss, but this is not sustainable or practical and leaves individuals fatigued, irritable and disillusioned. Indeed, we saw from our case study that having a sensible approach to nutrition, not deprivation, and becoming more physically active at the same time, not only helped James to improve his body composition and energy levels, but also benefitted his performance.

Thus, the science tells us that diet is more important than exercise when it comes to weight loss – this is because physical activity stimulates appetite. However, without exercise, you can't maintain your weight loss, as you need the gains in lean muscle mass as a response to training, to help keep metabolism high.

We know from our section on RED-S that it's a fine line; if you create too big a deficit through restrictive eating and high training load, you put the body in more stress and thus it down-regulates biological function, leading to deteriorations in both health and performance. But equally, the *BMJ* 2020 study shows us that diet alone is not sufficient to cause and maintain weight loss, so how can we strike the right balance?

The key is probably not to focus on achieving a specific weight, or encouraging dietary rules. The literature tells us that it is better to consider lifestyle in general, changing certain sustainable behaviours and making the outcome based on health parameters, rather than the number on the scales. Remember, weight tells us very little about the individual, from their personality to their actual body composition. We know that muscle has a higher mass than fat but takes up less room, which is why many people may see changes in girth measurements but not numbers on the scale.

Before embarking on any weight-loss plan, it is worth taking the time to consider if it is absolutely necessary – are you legitimately overweight and is this having an impact on your health? If you are active, eat well and have low risk of disease related to being overweight, but the number on the scales is not ideal, then trying to change anything further may not be to your benefit. However, if you are carrying a few extra pounds and/or have been told by your GP that your cholesterol and blood pressure are a bit high, then making some lifestyle changes around nutrition and exercise will help, but this doesn't mean you have to take things to the extreme.

We know that the most sustainable weight-loss approaches involve a deficit of no more than 100 calories a day and entail both making nutrient-dense choices and becoming more physically active. The present guidelines recommend 150 minutes a week, and this can be walking – it doesn't mean you need to take up extreme sport.

When it comes to athletes, the situation can be complicated. Very few athletes need to lose weight, but the culture within sport often blurs these lines. There is a big difference between body mass and body composition. An athlete with a higher lean muscle mass will probably weigh more than one with more body fat, and yet the 'lighter makes you faster' mentality is still rife, particularly in sports where power-to-weight ratio is a focus, such as endurance or climbing. When you talk to the most successful and sustainable athletes, they never put this down to their weight. They attribute their consistency and performances to sufficient and appropriate fuelling to support their training load, the right training for their outcome and adequate rest.

That said, in some sports and with some athletes, at certain times, it may be appropriate to try and improve body composition. A leaner body tends to be powerful and can create more force and speed.

Contrary to what many might believe, achieving a leaner body is not about restrictive practices or removing food groups. Remember that low-carbohydrate, high-fat diets have a negative effect on performance economy, so even if you did become a few per cent leaner, performance would still be compromised. The best way to achieve a leaner composition is to actually move more and eat more, so that your requirements match your training and your body has the energy to adapt from the training stimulus.

There is a place for weight loss, but it needs to be managed appropriately. In those who would benefit from losing weight to improve health parameters and metrics, making sustainable lifestyle changes should be the focus. This might simply mean swapping full-sugar drinks for no-added-sugar versions to start with, or trying to take the stairs at work rather than the lift.

In athletes, care needs to be taken so that the focus is body composition rather than mass.

How do you know what does work?

The one thing I hope you have taken from this book is that no one size fits all. Genetics, physiology, gender, ethnic background, training age and actual age all have an influence, which means care needs to be taken when starting on a new approach to nutrition based on an article you have read, hearsay or even your own research. Good scientific evidence with robust studies helps us to develop guidelines and recommendations, but the true art to knowing what works for you is trial and error.

All the way through the book, we have spoken about the importance of considering the purpose behind changing your nutritional approach. Once you are confident that you have armed yourself with the appropriate information and are aware of any potential risks, it is the right time to embark on something different. However, how do you then know it is working for you?

One of the criticisms I have about a lot of the nutrition trends that seem to take the world by storm is the fact that we often haven't seen the longitudinal data or outcome, but the media has got hold of some preliminary results and created a sensationalist headline.

An example that came about just this week of writing is the claim that we should all be able to fit into the same jeans size as we did when we were twenty-one years old, as this will reduce our risk of type 2 diabetes. The study has been commissioned by Diabetes UK and, while the results will no doubt be of interest, the *Guardian* made this a headline story when the reality is that the study is still in its infancy and the data won't be made available for two years.

We have already seen that many of the studies done on the low-carbohydrate, high-fat approach were too short to appreciate the full impact this approach has on someone's health and performance, but, equally, should you wait two years if there are some suggestions that the particular nutritional strategy you have undertaken may not be working for you?

Of course not. While it may take two years before you see any potential negative consequences, three to six months is a good amount of time to see if a new approach is making a positive difference.

On the whole, how you feel and your physical performance is a good indicator that your training and nutritional approach is working for you. Keep a training diary, logging your diet, training, sleep and how you feel, to monitor long-term trends. Remember, having a couple of bad days probably doesn't mean anything, but a couple of bad weeks is an indicator that something isn't right and needs to change.

In these cases, blood testing may be appropriate to identify potential underlying causes. My biochemistry and clinical background in nutrition has always meant that I have a real interest in what's going on within the body. For this reason, I'm a big fan of monitoring biomarkers – or more simply put, blood values of key markers, such as iron, vitamin D and hormones, that can tell us about immune, bone and hormonal health, inflammation and thus readiness to train and compete. The best time to consider monitoring bloods would be if you are starting to notice prolonged fatigue that you can't shift through resting, poor adaptation to training and poor recovery between training sessions.

Blood tests are very useful, but they can be hard to justify and most likely won't be available on the NHS. That said, there are numerous private biomarker companies that now offer finger-prick testing specifically with your performance and health in mind. I personally use Forth Edge and check the above markers at least twice a year, especially as I've got older.

Monitoring your sleep, motivation to train, energy levels, recovery between training sessions and then general adaptation to training and progression is also very useful and can highlight if something is a little off-kilter.

The best advice I can give, though, is not to be fearful of stopping an approach. Remember that our bodies are complex and hugely influenced by our genetics, lifestyle and environments. It's not a failing if the latest trend doesn't work for you, it's just understanding that your body has requirements that need to be met. In the same way, we may also find that what once worked for us no longer does, but learning to respond to your body's needs is an important part of being human. Where I think it can be harder is when the way you want to eat is based on some of your core values. I believe in this situation it is best to try and find the pivot point of how far you can follow an approach that aligns with your values and moral standards balanced with what is best for your health and performance.

The final word

Nutrition is not rocket science; however, nutrition is complex. While it should be about personal preference, we have uncovered that food choice is multifactorial and has numerous influences, from your cultural and educational background to medical and clinical needs, socio-economic status and popular science.

When working with athletes, there is nutrition for health and then there is nutrition for performance, and at times these are not compatible. For example, endurance athletes who do long- and ultra-distance sportive will need to consume a large amount of sugar to meet their fuelling requirements at certain times, which doesn't align with present public health guidelines. This doesn't make athletes unhealthy; on the contrary, it demonstrates the importance of an adaptive and flexible approach to achieve optimal performance.

Athletes need to take care that they don't let their hunger for success and performance blur lines, as this can lead to nutritional beliefs and behaviours that may not be appropriate or helpful.

Regardless of whether you are an athlete, a weekend warrior, someone new to exercise or just interested in the science behind the latest nutritional approaches, one thing to remember is:

Health is an attitude that encompasses total embodiment; that is mind and body.

Health and healthy eating is not a list of good or bad foods; it's not consuming a long line of novel ingredients and supplements; it's not about the training you do or the way your body looks.

We are a society that is driven by image, but by creating these body ideals we lose sight of what really makes us happy.

Social comparison will never fulfil you or provide you with joy. Just because a person's body looks a certain way, or they have a particular job or they have achieved a sporting outcome to which they aspired, doesn't make them any more accepted or loved. They would be the same person without all those disguises. This is just the narrative we have created.

For me, food is more than what it says about me. It is a chance to connect with those I love. It is an opportunity to learn about new cultures. It is a practice that feeds into my well-being, whether that is through the foods I eat and the associations they have or from sharing a plate, which is central to good chat and laughter.

While many struggle with understanding balance, moderation is exactly this: where no foods are off limits, where you tune into your internal cues and know when you are satisfied. It is about understanding that the body doesn't keep a daily tally and therefore overcompensating is not necessary, but trusting that if you listen, your body will tell you what you need. All too often when we restrict or deprive, this is when our body and brain becomes fixated on food and we lose sight of what we really need.

While certain nutritional practices work for some, they may be detrimental to others. Whatever your chosen path with nutrition, always try to have an open mind and monitor how your body is feeling, recovering and responding. A particular approach may work for a while, but it may not be the best practice forever. Tuning in, listening and being aware of some of the potential risks will ensure that you maintain optimal health and, thus, performance.

One final point: remember that the human body is made up of a series of feedback loops which makes it good at regulation, especially when we nurture and nourish it appropriately.

A healthy body and mind

Healthy hormones

Healthy body

Energy in

Energy out

ACKNOWLEDGEMENTS

Firstly, a huge thank you to everyone at Vertebrate for believing in me and this book. A special thanks to Kirsty for asking me to write the book and then continuing to hold my hand through the process.

A massive thanks to Jen Benson, someone I'm lucky to call my friend and who I have shared many miles with on the trails putting the world to rights. Jen did the main edits to this book and without her support, care and invested interest, I would still be writing this book. Writing a book is hard work, but being an editor and friend to the author is probably harder. I can't think of anyone I would rather trust and who I have the utmost respect for to help me get this book right and give it the platform it deserves. Thank you, Jen. I hope you are as proud of this book as I am.

Writing is a journey. One that takes you to all sorts of places – sometimes you get lost in the words you are writing, and at other times you wait for the right words to appear. It takes you through a roller coaster of emotions and no one can get through this without support. I am so lucky as I have a wonderful group of friends, my girls and not forgetting the two dogs, Bailey and Bosco, who keep me grounded, provide me with words of encouragement and continue to believe that my work is worth waiting for.

A special mention to Ewen, for always being there and creating a supportive environment that allows me to thrive – thank you, you really are the best.

To my girls, Maya and Ella, who are the reason I work so hard to show them that if you believe in yourself and stay determined, anything is possible, but who individually are shining bright.

To my good friend, running coach and fellow Vertebrate author Damian, for writing the foreword but also being a great sounding board.

I am incredibly grateful to all of you who agreed to be case studies in the book. Most of you, I am lucky to call friends, but all of you have made an impact in my working life in some way. Thank you for sharing your stories and helping to provide insight so we can collectively help so many others.

Finally, a big thanks to my team, who have been in the background, holding the fort and allowing me to have the time and space to create this book. You are all amazing and I feel so privileged watching you all grow and develop into the knowledgeable and caring professionals you all are.

NOTES

1. Hawkins, L.K., Farrow, C. & Thomas, J.M. (2020). 'Do perceived norms of social media users' eating habits and preferences predict our own food consumption and BMI?' *Appetite*, 149. https://doi.org/10.1016/j.appet.2020.104611

2. Shepherd, R. & Raats, M. (ed.) (2006). *The Psychology of Food Choice (Frontiers in Nutritional Science, No. 3)*. CABI Publishing. https://www.cabi.org/bookshop/book/9780851990323/

3. https://www.statista.com/statistics/1147773 average-annual-spending-on-health-and-fitness-supplements-in-selected-european-countries/

4. Jeukendrup, A.E., Rollo, I. & Carter, J.M. (2013). 'Carbohydrate mouth rinse: performance effects and mechanisms'. *Sports Science Exchange*. https://www.gssiweb.org/sports-science-exchange/article/sse-118-carbohydrate-mouth-rinse-performance-effects-and-mechanisms, accessed 25 March 2022.

5. Astrup, A., Magkos, F. et al. (2020). 'Saturated Fats and Health: A Reassessment and Proposal for Food-Based Recommendations: JACC State-of-the-Art Review'. *Journal of the American College of Cardiology*, 76(7), 844–857. https://doi.org/10.1016/j.jacc.2020.05.077

6. Trieu, K., Bhat, S., Dai, Z., Leander, K., Gigante, B., Qian, F. et al. (2021). 'Biomarkers of dairy fat intake, incident cardiovascular disease, and all-cause mortality: A cohort study, systematic review, and meta-analysis'. *PLOS Medicine*, 18(9): e1003763. https://doi.org/10.1371/journal.pmed.1003763

7.   'Food supplements'. https://www.food.gov.uk/business-guidance/
     food-supplements, accessed 25 March 2022.

8.   Michael, M.K., Joubert, L. & Witard, O.C. (2019). 'Assessment of
     Dietary Intake and Eating Attitudes in Recreational and Competitive
     Adolescent Rock Climbers: A Pilot Study'. *Frontiers in Nutrition*,
     Volume 6. https://doi.org/10.3389/fnut.2019.00064

9.   Nuffield Trust. 'Obesity'. https://www.nuffieldtrust.org.uk/resource/
     obesity, accessed 25 March 2022.

10. Health Survey for England (2019). 'Eating disorders'. http://
     healthsurvey.hscic.gov.uk/support-guidance/public-health/health-
     survey-for-england-2019/eating-disorders.aspx, accessed 25 March
     2022.

11. Statista. 'Diets and nutrition in the UK'. https://www.statista.com/
     forecasts/997894/diets-and-nutrition-in-the-uk, accessed 25 March
     2022.

12. National Diet and Nutrition Survey (NDNS). https://www.food.gov.
     uk/research/national-diet-and-nutrition-survey#:~:text=The%20
     National%20Diet%20and%20Nutrition,private%20households%20
     in%20the%20UK, accessed 25 March 2022.

13. Burke, L.M., Sharma, A.P., Heikura, I.A., Forbes, S.F., Holloway, M.,
     McKay, A.K.A. et al. (2020). 'Crisis of confidence averted:
     Impairment of exercise economy and performance in elite race
     walkers by ketogenic low carbohydrate, high fat (LCHF) diet is
     reproducible'. *PLOS ONE* 15(6): e0234027. https://doi.org/10.1371/
     journal.pone.0234027

14. Mata, F., Valenzuela, P.L., Gimenez, J., Tur, C., Ferreria, D.,
     Domínguez, R., Sanchez-Oliver, A.J. & Martínez Sanz, J.M. (2019).
     'Carbohydrate Availability and Physical Performance: Physiological
     Overview and Practical Recommendations'. *Nutrients*, 11(5), 1084.
     https://doi.org/10.3390/nu11051084

15. Hall, K.D. et al. (2021). 'Effect of a plant-based, low-fat diet versus an animal-based, ketogenic diet on ad libitum energy intake'. *Nature Medicine*, 27(2), 344–353. https://doi.org/10.1038/s41591-020-01209-1

16. Statista. 'Veganism and vegetarianism in the United Kingdom – statistics and facts'. https://www.statista.com/topics/7297/veganism-in-the-united-kingdom/, accessed 25 March 2022.

17. Vegan Society, 'Definition of veganism'. https://www.vegansociety.com/go-vegan/definition-veganism#:~:text=%22Veganism%20is%20a%20philosophy%20and,benefit%20of%20animals%2C%20humans%20and, accessed 25 March 2022.

18. Gary L. Francione. 'Vegan or Die: The Importance of Confronting Climate Change' (11 March 2019). https://gary-francione.medium.com/vegan-or-die-the-importance-of-confronting-climate-change-c08e31e56db8, accessed 9 March 2022.

19. Pelly, F.E. & Burkhart, S.J. (2014). 'Dietary regimens of athletes competing at the Delhi 2010 Commonwealth Games'. *International Journal of Sport Nutrition and Exercise Metabolism*, 24(1), 28–36. https://doi.org/10.1123/ijsnem.2013-0023

20. Vegan Society. 'What Every Vegan Should Know About Vitamin B12'. https://www.vegansociety.com/resources/nutrition-and-health/nutrients/vitamin-b12/what-every-vegan-should-know-about-vitamin-b12, accessed 25 March 2022.

21. Tong, T.Y.N., Appleby, P.N., Armstrong, M.E.G. et al. (2020). 'Vegetarian and vegan diets and risks of total and site-specific fractures: results from the prospective EPIC-Oxford study'. *BMC Medicine*, 18, 353. https://doi.org/10.1186/s12916-020-01815-3

22. Poore, J. & Nemecek, T. (2018). 'Reducing food's environmental impacts through producers and consumers'. *Science*, 360(6392), 987–992. https://doi.org/10.1126/science.aaq0216

23. Levy, E. & Chu, T. (2019). 'Intermittent Fasting and Its Effects on Athletic Performance: A Review.' *Current Sports Medicine Reports*, 18(7), 266–269. https://doi.org/10.1249/JSR.0000000000000614

24. Welton, S., Minty, R., O'Driscoll, T., Willms, H., Poirier, D., Madden, S. & Kelly, L. (2020). 'Intermittent fasting and weight loss: Systematic review.' *Canadian Family Physician/Le Médecin de Famille Canadien*, 66(2), 117–125.

25. Health Survey for England 2019. 'Overweight and obesity in adults and children.' https://files.digital.nhs.uk/9D/4195D5/HSE19-Overweight-obesity-rep.pdf, accessed 25 March 2022.

26. Sport England. 'Active Lives Adult Survey May 2019/20 Report.' https://sportengland-production-files.s3.eu-west-2.amazonaws.com/s3fs-public/2020-10/Active%20Lives%20Adult%20May%2019-20%20Report.pdf?VersionId=AYzBswpBmlh9cNcH8TFctPI38v4Ok2JD, accessed 25 March 2022.

27. Statista. 'Number of women who participated in sport and physical activity at least twice in the last 28 days in England from 2016 to 2021.' https://www.statista.com/statistics/1024168/female-sport-physical-activity-participation-england, accessed 25 March 2022.

28. TCS London Marathon. 'World Record for 2020 London Marathon.' https://www.tcslondonmarathon.com/news-and-media/latest-news/world-record-for-2020-london-marathon, accessed 25 March 2022.

29. Carmichael, M.A., Thomson, R.L., Moran, L.J. & Wycherley, T.P. (2021). 'The Impact of Menstrual Cycle Phase on Athletes' Performance: A Narrative Review.' *International Journal of Environmental Research and Public Health*, 18(4), 1667. https://doi.org/10.3390/ijerph18041667

30. Harris, J.E., Pinckard, K.M., Wright, K.R. et al. (2020). 'Exercise-induced 3'-sialyllactose in breast milk is a critical mediator to improve metabolic health and cardiac function in mouse offspring.' *Nature Metabolism*, 2, 678–687. https://doi.org/10.1038/s42255-020-0223-8

31. NICE (National Institute for Health and Care Excellence). 'Menopause: diagnosis and management'. https://www.nice.org.uk/ guidance/ng23/resources menopause-diagnosis-and-management-pdf-1837330217413

32. Bailey, T.G., Cable, N.T., Aziz, N., Atkinson, G., Cuthbertson, D.J., Low, D.A. & Jones, H. (2016). 'Exercise training reduces the acute physiological severity of post-menopausal hot flushes'. *The Journal of Physiology*, 594(3), 657–667. https://doi.org/10.1113/JP271456

33. Mishra, N., Mishra, V.N. & Devanshi (2011). 'Exercise beyond menopause: Dos and Don'ts'. *Journal of Mid-Life Health*, 2(2), 51–56. https://doi.org/10.4103/0976-7800.92524

34. United Nations. 'Global Issues: Ageing'. https://www.un.org/en/ global-issues/ageing, accessed 25 March 2022.

35. Petermann-Rocha, F., Ferguson, L.D., Gray, S.R., Rodríguez-Gómez, I., Sattar, N., Siebert, S., Ho, F.K., Pell, J.P. & Celis-Morales, C. (2021). 'Association of sarcopenia with incident osteoporosis: a prospective study of 168,682 UK biobank participants'. *Journal of Cachexia, Sarcopenia and Muscle*, 12(5), 1179–1188. https://doi.org/10.1002/ jcsm.12757

36. Trappe, S.W., Costill, D.L., Vukovich, M.D., Jones, J. & Melham, T. (1996). 'Aging among elite distance runners: a 22-yr longitudinal study'. *Journal of Applied Physiology*, 80(1), 285–290. https://doi. org/10.1152/jappl.1996.80.1.285

37. Figel, K., Pritchett, K., Pritchett, R. & Broad, E. (2018). 'Energy and Nutrient Issues in Athletes with Spinal Cord Injury: Are They at Risk for Low Energy Availability?' *Nutrients*, 10(8), 1078. https://doi. org/10.3390/nu10081078

38. Ge, L., Sadeghirad, B., Ball, G.D.C., da Costa, B.R., Hitchcock, C.L., Svendrovski, A. et al. (2020). 'Comparison of dietary macronutrient patterns of 14 popular named dietary programmes for weight and cardiovascular risk factor reduction in adults: systematic review and network meta-analysis of randomised trials'. *BMJ* 2020; 369:m696. https://doi.org/10.1136/bmj.m696

BIBLIOGRAPHY AND REFERENCES

Journals

Ackerman, K.E., Singhal, V., Baskaran, C., Slattery, M., Campoverde Reyes, K.J., Toth, A., Eddy, K.T., Bouxsein, M.L., Lee, H., Klibanski, A. & Misra, M. (2019). 'Oestrogen replacement improves bone mineral density in oligo-amenorrhoeic athletes: a randomised clinical trial'. *British Journal of Sports Medicine*, 53(4), 229–236. https://doi.org/10.1136/bjsports-2018-099723

Bailey, A. (2009). 'Menopause and physical fitness'. *Menopause*, 16(5), 856–857. https://doi.org/10.1097/gme.0b013e3181b0d018

Barnes, K.R. & Kilding, A.E. (2015). 'Running economy: measurement, norms, and determining factors'. *Sports Med – Open*, 1(8). https://doi.org/10.1186/s40798-015-0007-y

Burke, L.M. (2015). 'Re-Examining High-Fat Diets for Sports Performance: Did We Call the "Nail in the Coffin" Too Soon?' *Sports Medicine* (Auckland, N.Z.), 45, Supplement 1, S33–S49. https://doi.org/10.1007/s40279-015-0393-9

Burke, L.M. (2020). 'Ketogenic low-CHO, high-fat diet: the future of elite endurance sport?' *The Journal of Physiology*, 599(3), 819–843. https://doi.org/10.1113/JP278928

Burke, L.M. & Hawley, J.A. (2018). 'Swifter, higher, stronger: What's on the menu?' *Science* (New York, N.Y.), 362(6416), 781–787. https://doi.org/10.1126/science.aau2093

Burke, L.M., Angus, D.J., Cox, G.R., Cummings, N.K., Febbraio, M.A., Gawthorn, K., Hawley, J.A., Minehan, M., Martin, D.T. & Hargreaves, M. (2000). 'Effect of fat adaptation and carbohydrate restoration on metabolism and performance during prolonged cycling'. *Journal of Applied Physiology* (Bethesda, Md.: 1985), 89(6), 2413–2421. https://doi.org/10.1152/jappl.2000.89.6.2413

Burke, L.M., Close, G.L., Lundy, B., Mooses, M., Morton, J.P. & Tenforde, A.S. (2018). 'Relative Energy Deficiency in Sport in Male Athletes: A Commentary on Its Presentation Among Selected Groups of Male Athletes'. *International Journal of Sport Nutrition and Exercise Metabolism*, 28(4), 364–374. https://doi.org/10.1123/ijsnem.2018-0182

Burke, L.M., Ross, M.L., Garvican-Lewis, L.A., Welvaert, M., Heikura, I.A., Forbes, S.G., Mirtschin, J.G., Cato, L.E., Strobel, N., Sharma, A.P. & Hawley, J.A. (2017). 'Low carbohydrate, high fat diet impairs exercise economy and negates the performance benefit from intensified training in elite race walkers'. *The Journal of Physiology*, 595(9), 2785–2807. https://doi.org/10.1113/JP273230

Burke, L.M., Whitfield, J., Heikura, I.A., Ross, M., Tee, N., Forbes, S.F., Hall, R., McKay, A., Wallett, A.M. & Sharma, A.P. (2021). 'Adaptation to a low carbohydrate high fat diet is rapid but impairs endurance exercise metabolism and performance despite enhanced glycogen availability'. *The Journal of Physiology*, 599(3), 771–790. https://doi.org/10.1113/JP280221

Desbrow, B., Burd, N.A., Tarnopolsky, M., Moore, D.R. & Elliott-Sale, K.J. (2019). 'Nutrition for Special Populations: Young, Female, and Masters Athletes'. *International Journal of Sport Nutrition and Exercise Metabolism*, 29(2), 220–227. https://doi.org/10.1123/ijsnem.2018-0269

Figel, K., Pritchett, K., Pritchett, R. & Broad, E. (2018). 'Energy and Nutrient Issues in Athletes with Spinal Cord Injury: Are They at Risk for Low Energy Availability?' *Nutrients*, 10(8), 1078. https://doi.org/10.3390/nu10081078

Firth, J., Torous, J., Stubbs, B., Firth, J.A., Steiner, G.Z., Smith, L., Alvarez-Jimenez, M., Gleeson, J., Vancampfort, D., Armitage, C.J. & Sarris, J. (2019). 'The "online brain": how the Internet may be changing our cognition'. *World Psychiatry: official journal of the World Psychiatric Association (WPA)*, 18(2), 119–129. https://doi.org/10.1002/wps.20617

Gaesser, G. (2015). 'Carbohydrates, performance and weight loss: Is low the way to go or the way to bonk?' *Agro Food Industry Hi-Tech*, 26(6), 35–38.

Ge, L., Sadeghirad, B., Ball, G.D.C., da Costa, B.R., Hitchcock, C.L., Svendrovski, A. et al. (2020). 'Comparison of dietary macronutrient patterns of 14 popular named dietary programmes for weight and cardiovascular risk factor reduction in adults: systematic review and network meta-analysis of randomised trials'. *British Medical Journal* 2020;369:m696. https://doi.org/10.1136/bmj.m696

Goedecke, J.H., Christie, C., Wilson, G., Dennis, S.C., Noakes, T.D., Hopkins, W.G. & Lambert, E.V. (1999). 'Metabolic adaptations to a high-fat diet in endurance cyclists'. *Metabolism: Clinical and Experimental*, 48(12), 1509–1517. https://doi.org/10.1016/s0026-0495(99)90238-x

Gordon, C.M., Ackerman, K.E., Berga, S.L., Kaplan, J.R., Mastorakos, G., Misra, M., Murad, M.H., Santoro, N.F. & Warren, M.P. (2017). 'Functional Hypothalamic Amenorrhea: An Endocrine Society Clinical Practice Guideline'. *The Journal of Clinical Endocrinology & Metabolism*, 102(5), 1413–1439. https://doi.org/10.1210/jc.2017-00131

Hall, K.D., Guo, J., Courville, A.B. et al. (2021). 'Effect of a plant-based, low-fat diet versus an animal-based, ketogenic diet on ad libitum energy intake'. *Nature Medicine*, 27, 344–353. https://doi.org/10.1038/s41591-020-01209-1

Hilton, L.K. & Loucks, A.B. (2000). 'Low energy availability, not exercise stress, suppresses the diurnal rhythm of leptin in healthy young women'. *American Journal of Physiology*. Endocrinology and Metabolism, 278(1), E43–E49. https://doi.org/10.1152/ajpendo.2000.278.1.E43

173

Hinman, S.K., Smith, K.B., Quillen, D.M. & Smith, M.S. (2015). 'Exercise in Pregnancy: A Clinical Review'. *Sports Health*, 7(6), 527–531. https://doi.org/10.1177/1941738115599358

Kortetmäki, T. & Oksanen, M. (2020). 'Is there a convincing case for climate veganism?' *Agriculture and Human Values*, 38, 729–740 (2021). https://doi.org/10.1007/s10460-020-10182-x

Lambert, E.V., Speechly, D.P., Dennis, S.C. & Noakes, T.D. (1994). 'Enhanced endurance in trained cyclists during moderate intensity exercise following 2 weeks adaptation to a high fat diet'. *European Journal of Applied Physiology and Occupational Physiology*, 69(4), 287–293. https://doi.org/10.1007/BF00392032

Levy, E. & Chu, T. (2019). 'Intermittent Fasting and Its Effects on Athletic Performance: A Review'. *Current Sports Medicine Reports*, 18(7), 266–269. https://doi.org/10.1249/JSR.0000000000000614

Logue, D.M., Madigan, S.M., Melin, A., Delahunt, E., Heinen, M., Donnell, S.M. & Corish, C.A. (2020). 'Low Energy Availability in Athletes 2020: An Updated Narrative Review of Prevalence, Risk, Within-Day Energy Balance, Knowledge, and Impact on Sports Performance'. *Nutrients*, 12(3), 835. https://doi.org/10.3390/nu12030835

Louis, J., Vercruyssen, F., Dupuy, O. & Bernard, T. (2019). 'Nutrition for Master Athletes: Is There a Need for Specific Recommendations?' *Journal of Aging and Physical Activity*, 28(3), 489–498. Advance online publication. https://doi.org/10.1123/japa.2019-0190

Manore, M.M. (2005). 'Exercise and the Institute of Medicine recommendations for nutrition'. *Current Sports Medicine Reports*, 4(4), 193–198. https://doi.org/10.1097/01.csmr.0000306206.72186.00

Martinelli, P.M., Sorpreso, I.C.E., Raimundo, R.D., Junior, O. de S.L., Zangirolami-Raimundo, J., Malveira de Lima, M.V. et al. (2020). 'Heart rate variability helps to distinguish the intensity of menopausal symptoms: A prospective, observational and transversal study'. *PLOS ONE*, 15(1): e0225866. https://doi.org/10.1371/journal.pone.0225866

Mata, F., Valenzuela, P.L., Gimenez, J., Tur, C., Ferreria, D., Domínguez, R., Sanchez-Oliver, A.J. & Martínez Sanz, J.M. (2019). 'Carbohydrate Availability and Physical Performance: Physiological Overview and Practical Recommendations'. *Nutrients*, 11(5), 1084. https://doi.org/10.3390/nu11051084

Meignié, A., Duclos, M., Carling, C., Orhant, E., Provost, P., Toussaint, J.F. & Antero, J. (2021). 'The Effects of Menstrual Cycle Phase on Elite Athlete Performance: A Critical and Systematic Review'. *Frontiers in Physiology*, 12. https://doi.org/10.3389/fphys.2021.654585

Michael, M.K., Joubert, L. & Witard, O.C. (2019). 'Assessment of Dietary Intake and Eating Attitudes in Recreational and Competitive Adolescent Rock Climbers: A Pilot Study'. *Frontiers in Nutrition*, 6. https://doi.org/10.3389/fnut.2019.00064

Mishra, N., Mishra, V.N. & Devanshi (2011). 'Exercise beyond menopause: Dos and Don'ts'. *Journal of Mid-Life Health*, 2(2), 51–56. https://doi.org/10.4103/0976-7800.92524

Moore, D.R., Churchward-Venne, T.A., Witard, O., Breen, L., Burd, N.A., Tipton, K.D. & Phillips, S.M. (2015). 'Protein ingestion to stimulate myofibrillar protein synthesis requires greater relative protein intakes in healthy older versus younger men'. *The Journals of Gerontology. Series A: Biological Sciences and Medical Sciences*, 70(1), 57–62. https://doi.org/10.1093/gerona/glu103

Mountjoy, M., Sundgot-Borgen, J.K., Burke, L.M. et al. (2018). 'IOC consensus statement on relative energy deficiency in sport (RED-S): 2018 update'. *British Journal of Sports Medicine*, 52: 687–697. http://dx.doi.org/10.1136/bjsports-2018-099193

Mountjoy, M., Sundgot-Borgen, J., Burke, L., Carter, S., Constantini, N., Lebrun, C., Meyer, N., Sherman, R., Steffen, K., Budgett, R., Ljungqvist, A. & Ackerman, K. (2015). 'RED-S CAT. Relative Energy Deficiency in Sport (RED-S) Clinical Assessment Tool (CAT)'. *British Journal of Sports Medicine*, 49(7), 421–423. https://doi.org/10.1136/bjsports-2015-094873

Mountjoy, M., Sundgot-Borgen, J.K., Burke, L.M., Ackerman, K.E., Blauwet, C., Constantini, N., Lebrun, C., Lundy, B., Melin, A.K., Meyer, N.L., Sherman, R.T., Tenforde, A.S., Klungland Torstveit, M. & Budgett, R. (2018). 'IOC consensus statement on relative energy deficiency in sport (RED-S): 2018 update'. *British Journal of Sports Medicine*, 52(11), 687–697. https://doi.org/10.1136/bjsports-2018-099193

Murray, B. & Rosenbloom, C. (2018). 'Fundamentals of glycogen metabolism for coaches and athletes'. *Nutrition Reviews*, 76(4), 243–259. https://doi.org/10.1093/nutrit/nuy001

O'Keeffe, K.A., Keith, R.E., Wilson, G.D. & Blessing, D.L. (1989). 'Dietary carbohydrate intake and endurance exercise performance of trained female cyclists'. *Nutrition Research*, 9(8), 819–830.

Otis, C.L., Drinkwater, B., Johnson, M., Loucks, A. & Wilmore, J. (1997). 'American College of Sports Medicine position stand. The Female Athlete Triad'. *Medicine and Science in Sports and Exercise*, 29(5), i–ix. https://doi.org/10.1097/00005768-199705000-00037

Paoli, A., Grimaldi, K., D'Agostino, D., Cenci, L., Moro, T., Bianco, A. & Palma, A. (2012). 'Ketogenic diet does not affect strength performance in elite artistic gymnasts'. *Journal of the International Society of Sports Nutrition*, 9(1), 34. https://doi.org/10.1186/1550-2783-9-34

Peos, J.J., Norton, L.E., Helms, E.R., Galpin, A.J. & Fournier, P. (2019). 'Intermittent Dieting: Theoretical Considerations for the Athlete'. *Sports* (Basel, Switzerland), 7(1), 22. https://doi.org/10.3390/sports7010022

Phinney, S.D., Bistrian, B.R., Evans, W.J., Gervino, E. & Blackburn, G.L. (1983). 'The human metabolic response to chronic ketosis without caloric restriction: preservation of submaximal exercise capability with reduced carbohydrate oxidation'. *Metabolism: Clinical and Experimental*, 32(8), 769–776. https://doi.org/10.1016/0026-0495(83)90106-3

Rogerson, D. (2017). 'Vegan diets: practical advice for athletes and exercisers'. *Journal of the International Society of Sports Nutrition*, 14(36). https://doi.org/10.1186/s12970-017-0192-9

Rossato, L.T., Schoenfeld, B.J. & de Oliveira, E.P. (2020). 'Is there sufficient evidence to supplement omega-3 fatty acids to increase muscle mass and strength in young and older adults?' *Clinical Nutrition*, 39(1), 23–32. https://doi.org/10.1016/j.clnu.2019.01.001

Rymer, J., Brian, K., Regan, L. (2019). 'HRT and breast cancer risk'. *BMJ* 2019; 367:l5928. https://doi.org/10.1136/bmj.l5928

Rynders, C.A., Thomas, E.A., Zaman, A., Pan, Z., Catenacci, V.A. & Melanson, E.L. (2019). 'Effectiveness of Intermittent Fasting and Time-Restricted Feeding Compared to Continuous Energy Restriction for Weight Loss'. *Nutrients*, 11(10), 2442. https://doi.org/10.3390/nu11102442

Santoro, N. (2016). 'Perimenopause: From Research to Practice'. *Journal of Women's Health*, 25(4), 332–339. https://doi.org/10.1089/jwh.2015.5556

Slater, J., McLay-Cooke, R., Brown, R. & Black, K. (2016). 'Female Recreational Exercisers at Risk for Low Energy Availability'. *International Journal of Sport Nutrition and Exercise Metabolism*, 26(5), 421–427. https://doi.org/10.1123/ijsnem.2015-0245

Sternfeld, B. & Dugan, S. (2011). 'Physical activity and health during the menopausal transition'. *Obstetrics and Gynecology Clinics of North America*, 38(3), 537–566. https://doi.org/10.1016/j.ogc.2011.05.008

Stockman, M.C., Thomas, D., Burke, J. & Apovian, C.M. (2018). 'Intermittent Fasting: Is the Wait Worth the Weight?' *Current Obesity Reports*, 7(2), 172–185. https://doi.org/10.1007/s13679-018-0308-9

Sutton, E.F., Beyl, R., Early, K.S., Cefalu, W., Ravussin, E. & Peterson, C.M. (2018). 'Early Time-Restricted Feeding Improves Insulin Sensitivity, Blood Pressure, and Oxidative Stress Even without Weight Loss in Men with Prediabetes'. *Cell Metabolism*, 27(6), 1212–1221. https://doi.org/10.1016/j.cmet.2018.04.010

Thomas, D.T., Erdman, K.A. & Burke, L.M. (2016). 'Position of the Academy of Nutrition and Dietetics, Dietitians of Canada, and the American College of Sports Medicine: Nutrition and Athletic Performance'. *Journal of the Academy of Nutrition and Dietetics*, 116(3), 501–528. https://doi.org/10.1016/j.jand.2015.12.006

Thurecht, R. & Pelly, F. (2020). 'Key Factors Influencing the Food Choices of Athletes at Two Distinct Major International Competitions'. *Nutrients*, 12(4), 924. https://doi.org/10.3390/nu12040924

Torstveit, M.K., Fahrenholtz, I.L., Lichtenstein, M.B. et al. (2019). 'Exercise dependence, eating disorder symptoms and biomarkers of Relative Energy Deficiency in Sports (RED-S) among male endurance athletes'. *BMJ Open Sport & Exercise Medicine*, 2019(5): e000439. https://doi.org/10.1136/bmjsem-2018-000439

Vitale, K. & Hueglin, S. (2021). 'Update on vegetarian and vegan athletes: a review'. *The Journal of Physical Fitness and Sports Medicine*, 10, 1–11. https://doi.org/10.7600/jpfsm.10.1

Williams, N.I., Mallinson, R.J. & De Souza, M.J. (2019). 'Rationale and study design of an intervention of increased energy intake in women with exercise-associated menstrual disturbances to improve menstrual function and bone health: The REFUEL study'. *Contemporary Clinical Trials Communications*, 14. https://doi.org/10.1016/j.conctc.2019.100325

Wirnitzer, K.C. (2020). 'Vegan Diet in Sports and Exercise – Health Benefits and Advantages to Athletes and Physically Active People: A Narrative Review'. *International Journal of Sports and Exercise Medicine*, 6:165. https://doi.org/10.23937/2469-5718/1510165

Websites, blogs and guidelines

Akers, W. (14 November 2019). 'Elite Athletes Are Going Vegan. Will It Help You?' https://www.healthline.com/health-news/pro-athletes-are-going-vegan-will-it-help-2

BBC Wales (22 September 2015). 'Black and ethnic minorities face barriers to sport, report says'. https://www.bbc.co.uk/news/uk-wales-34324066

Bean, A. (9 November 2020). 'Will a Plant-Based Diet Make You a Better Athlete?' https://anitabean.co.uk/will-a-plant-based-diet-make-you-a-better-athlete/

Clark, N. (10 December 2020). 'Is the lighter athlete the better athlete?' https://nancyclarkrd.com/2020/12/10/is-the-lighter-athlete-the-better-athlete/

Collins, K. & Klemm, S. (6 June 2021). 'Breastfeeding and the Athlete'. https://www.eatright.org/health/pregnancy/breast-feeding/breastfeeding-and-the-athlete

Eckert, R. 'Low vs. High Carbohydrate Diets for Endurance Performance'. https://www.trainingpeaks.com/blog/low-vs-high-carbohydrate-diet-endurance/

Equality in Sport. 'Ethnic Minority Communities and Sport'. https://equalityinsport.org/wp-content/uploads/2015/12/bmebackground2002.pdf

Hamilton, A. 'Master Athletes: how to maintain endurance fitness as the years tick by', Sports Performance Bulletin. https://www.sportsperformancebulletin.com/endurance-training/masters/endurance-training-master-athletes/

Harvard Health Publishing (1 December 2021). 'Heart rate variability: How it might indicate well-being'. https://www.health.harvard.edu/blog/heart-rate-variability-new-way-track-well-2017112212789

Johns Hopkins Medicine. 'Nutrition During Pregnancy'. https://www.hopkinsmedicine.org/health/wellness-and-prevention-nutrition-during-pregnancy

NICE (National Institute for Health and Care Excellence, 12 November 2015). 'Menopause: diagnosis and management', NG23. https://www.nice.org.uk/guidance/ng23/resourcesmenopause-diagnosis-and-management-pdf-1837330217413

NICE (National Institute for Health and Care Excellence). 'Management of secondary amenorrhoea'. https://cks.nice.org.uk/topics/amenorrhoea/management/secondary-amenorrhoea/

Open University, OpenLearn (updated 23 June 2020). 'Black lives matter in sport too: what is the BAME experience of sport in the UK?' https://www.open.edu/openlearn/health-sports-psychology/sport-fitness/black-lives-matter-sport-too-what-the-bame-experience-sport-the-uk

paralympic.org (24 August 2021). 'Tokyo 2020 sets the record for most athletes and women at a Paralympic Games'. https://www.paralympic.org/news/tokyo-2020-sets-record-most-athletes-and-women-paralympic-games

Science Daily (29 June 2020). 'Study finds exercise increases benefits of breast milk for babies'. https://www.sciencedaily.com/releases/2020/06/200629120220.htm

Sherrell, Z. 'What to know about social media and mental health'. https://www.medicalnewstoday.com/articles/social-media-and-mental-health

Sport England. 'Getting people in ethnic groups active'. https://www.sportengland.org/know-your-audience/demographic-knowledge/ethnicity?section=getting_people_in_ethnic_groups_active

Tello, M. (16 November 2021). 'Intermittent fasting: Surprising update'. https://www.health.harvard.edu/blog/intermittent-fasting-surprising-update-2018062914156

Tousignant, Dr K. (27 July 2021). 'What science says about intermittent fasting and the gut microbiome'. https://insight.microba.com/blog/what-science-says-about-intermittent-fasting-and-the-gut-microbiome/

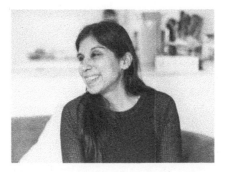

ABOUT THE AUTHOR

Renee McGregor is a leading sports and eating disorder specialist dietitian with twenty years' experience working in clinical and performance nutrition. She has worked with athletes across the globe, including supporting Olympic (London 2012), Paralympic (Rio 2016) and Commonwealth (Queensland 2018) teams. Renee also works closely with English and Scottish National Ballet, leading on their diet advisory and supporting dancers of all ages and abilities. She is regularly asked to work directly with high-performing and professional athletes who have developed a dysfunctional relationship with food that is impacting their performance, health and career.

Renee is also the founder of Team Renee McGregor, managing a team of practitioners specialising in supporting individuals and athletes of all levels and ages, coaches and sports science teams to provide nutritional strategies to enhance sports performance and manage eating disorders. This is reflected in her work on social media too, where she prides herself on proving an educational hub for both the professional and the everyday athlete.

Renee is a bestselling author of four books, including *Training Food* and *Orthorexia: When Healthy Eating Goes Bad*. When not inspiring others with her incredible work, Renee can be found running in the mountains and chasing the trails, most likely training for a crazy ultramarathon. In March 2022 she became British Trail Running champion for the short distance in the F45 category.